SMILE AT ME, DOCTOR

Joyce Delaney was born and brought up in Dublin. She qualified as a doctor at University College, Dublin, over twenty years ago and has worked in various branches of medicine ever since. She obtained a degree in Psychological Medicine in 1953 and is now on the staff of a large mental hospital in the north of England. She is the author of a novel, *Come Down from the Mountain*, and a contributor to many magazines, including *Nova* and *World Medicine*.

No Starch in my Coat, the first volume of her autobiography, is also published by Pan Books.

D1388490

By the same author in Pan Books

NO STARCH IN MY COAT

SMILE AT ME, DOCTOR

JOYCE DELANEY

PAN BOOKS LTD
LONDON AND SYDNEY

First published 1972 by Peter Davies Ltd
This edition published 1974 by Pan Books Ltd,
Cavaye Place, London SW10 9PG

ISBN 0 330 24095 1

*Printed and bound in England by
Hazell Watson & Viney Ltd,
Aylesbury, Bucks*

To Mark Barty-King

CHAPTER ONE

As you approach middle age, you expect to get into a rut. I'd decided I wasn't going to mind, but gradually the realization dawned that I could find myself a rut which paid better. So when I was offered an appointment at a hospital in the north of England, I didn't feel much doubt that I was doing the right thing in accepting. School fees were going to be a prominent item in my expenditure for the next few years; and although I wasn't unhappy at the Osbourne Hospital, there was little chance of getting a more lucrative job there. The hospital had moved forward, in that it now leaned heavily on female medical power, but the idea of women in more senior jobs still didn't go down very well.

'What's the name of the dump you're going to?' Dr Viney asked, on learning of my move. 'Bushy Park Hospital? Never heard of it, and God knows I know most of the bins in England. Where did you say it was? Haxton? A dreary place ... All slag heaps. Passed through it during the War.'

Viney looked blue with ill temper, and it couldn't have been because my leaving the Osbourne would inconvenience him. He'd been retired from the National Health Service for a number of years now, and lived in a kind of surly truce with his fat wife, in a large Victorian house with a lovely garden tended by Osbourne patients.

I used to visit Viney every two or three months and take him a bottle of wine. He liked to sup the warmed drink and extract every meaty bit of hospital gossip from me, which he then embellished with all sorts of scandalous surmises and fantasies. Cyanosed and gasping, he would cram his pipe into his mouth and chuckle over some really lurid tit-bit. It was probably my snippets of gossip and the memories I brought that he'd miss.

At a battle of the tongue it was impossible to beat Viney, and as he went on intoning his Dies Irae about my going north, I felt first a rising tide of impatience and then doubt.

Just like I'd felt before going to Malaya when the surgeon for whom I was then working had told me with a groan, 'You're mad, dear, mad. Think of the effect it will have on your complexion.'

"Ow do ... Fish-an'-chips ... Cloth-cap country ...' Viney recited. 'You're a donkey, Delaney, you really are. A perfectly good job here and you're galloping north.'

It was no use trying to explain *why* I was going: that I would be receiving a higher salary and thus getting a larger pension. Viney, probably because his wife had to work miracles with the small amount of money he gave her, thought that all women ought to be able to manage on a small wage. He chose to forget that I was what is rather oddly known in law as a 'feme-sole', and that whether or not my son ate properly depended on the sort of job I could get.

The older I grew, the more I blessed my father's hangover from the Famine, which made him see careers mainly from the salary angle. And he hadn't been wrong when he estimated that people would always need doctors. Another comforting thought had occurred to me one morning when I woke up and flexed my limbs with such difficulty that I longed for a squirt of oil in each joint: in an age where Youth was venerated, reaching forty meant plastic surgery if you could afford it and an apology if you couldn't. But people didn't mind their doctor having some lines and grey hairs, assuming (God bless them) that the physical evidence of mental fatigue must mean experience gained and thus a sounder diagnosis.

Viney's warnings and lamentations were depressing, but I had accepted the job after the interview and there was no going back. Anyway, all the doctors I used to know at the Osbourne had moved or left, and I didn't relish the thought of staying on as a sort of Oldest Inhabitant, hearing remarks like, 'Dr Delaney remembers the Insulin Treatment, you know,' and seeing the awed goggle of some newly qualified whizz-kid. Insulin therapy, once used in the treatment of schizophrenia, was discarded in the 1940s, and for a doctor to remember using it was like a Chelsea pensioner recalling Mafeking!

No, the slower tempo of life in the north would ease the

necessary adjustment of nearing forty, and I visualized a more gracious passage through the sere and yellow of my life amidst the less hectic atmosphere of Bushy Park. Besides, when I'd visited the place I'd taken a liking to it. The grounds were splendid – it seemed that the head gardener had been in charge of a well-known duke's estate – and although the building itself, like all hospitals erected at the turn of the century, was solidly uncompromising outside, inside every effort had been made to make the place bright and cheerful. I'd noticed how happy some of the patients looked as they got ready for a trip to Blackpool, and there were far more nurses and ancillary staff than at the Osbourne.

Dr David Hedley, the Chairman of the Medical Advisory Board, was waiting for me in his room on my first day at Bushy Park. He was a small twinkling man with a shiny bald head and equally bright blue eyes. His suit was brown and he reminded me of a small and kindly mole. After a few minutes of perfunctory chat about my journey north and whether my house was comfortable, he cleared his throat and told me that he hoped I wouldn't mind working with a woman doctor.

'For a start, anyway,' he added apologetically. 'Dr Sanders is – well, she's worked here for thirty years and we ... er ... we want her last year to ... well, not to be too strenuous for her.'

He didn't have to apologize. Hadn't I worked happily with Dr Ceri Thomas? I had no qualms about working under another female, and Dr Sanders seemed quite a character from what Hedley was saying. She'd come to Bushy Park not long after she qualified, had, Hedley told me, 'done the work of three doctors during the War', and even now devoted all her time and energy to the patients.

'Grand woman, Rose ... grand. Mind you, she has a bit of a temper, but then she's a redhead.'

Clearing his throat, he picked up the telephone and then thought better of it. Dr Sanders was 'a little impatient at times on the phone' and it might be better if I were to see her the following morning – he'd just remembered that today was her clinic day and she was always in a hurry on a Monday morning. Perhaps if I wouldn't mind slipping up to the ward that afternoon, the Sister would fill me in about things?

He was such a nice little man, Hedley, so obviously anxious to offend no one, that I was beginning to have my doubts about Dr Sanders. A first vision of a cosy silver-haired old campaigner was fading; the unwritten rule in hospitals was that the newcomer was always given the dirtiest jobs and the most difficult people to work with.

In spite of interruptions by frequent telephone calls and having to deal with a sheaf of letters brought in by a secretary, Dr Hedley managed to tell me about the routine at Bushy Park, which as far as I could tell didn't differ very much from the daily round at the Osbourne. The only change was that at Bushy Park I'd be doing even more out-patient work than at the Osbourne, and that, for a time, anyway, I'd be working with Dr Rose Sanders.

Rose was getting another big build-up – 'a heart of gold, Rose has ... a heart of gold' – when the door crashed open and in swept someone who looked like a fugitive from the Left Bank. She was about twenty-six, with a small compact body and a shock of brown hair that had been energetically streaked with gold. She wore no make-up except to outline her blue-green eyes, and her clothes looked as if they'd come from one of the seedier junk-shops. Her dark-green velvet suit was made for someone of nobler proportions, and she should have looked wrong but somehow didn't, probably because she wore it with such dash and *élan*. My impression of a rather wild Madonna faded, however, when she said, in a ripe Liverpudlian accent, 'I want to put in for me study leave, Dave. That bloody Board's never answered the letter I sent ...'

'Er – I'll look into it, Harriet. May I introduce Dr Delaney ... Dr Harriet Bentley.'

'Oh God! Me gear ...' I felt my hand gripped and met the flash of her enormous eyes before I had to bend to help her with the contents of her huge black shoulder-bag, which had spilled onto the carpet. There were pens, two worn-looking lipsticks and several objects whose use was a mystery to me, a few jotters and notebooks, a limp-looking package of crisps and a squashed-looking pound of sausages.

'I was wondering where the bangers had gone,' Harriet said, as she took the sausages from me.

As I got up, I saw Hedley glance at her with an expression midway between horror and fascination. Mrs Hedley was undoubtedly a tidy little soul who shopped at regular intervals and would never throw sausages absent-mindedly into her handbag, I reflected.

'I know what made me forget,' Harriet went on. 'I was on duty last night and I admitted a bloke into one of your wards, Dave. I think he's a Frohlichs Syndrome.'

'I wonder who you mean?'

'A short little guy with a red face and high blood-pressure. His name's Winters.'

'Oh, I know him. I saw him at the clinic. But I wouldn't have thought he was a Frohlichs, Harriet.'

'He is, because . . .'

Harriet launched into a fluent dissertation of why she thought the patient had this particular disease, which was caused by a glandular disturbance resulting in obesity and a red face. There was no doubt, I thought, listening to her, about this girl's intelligence quotient.

Another phone call gave Hedley the excuse I was sure he was looking for and I found myself being delivered to the care of Harriet Bentley for the morning.

'I know where we'll get a cuppa coffee. Come on, I had no breakfast because the bloody milkman left no milk. In here . . .'

Harriet swept me into a ward full of very old female patients. The Sister who tottered out to meet us was just as geriatric herself but from the way she gently dealt with the old ladies who interrupted us and saw them back to their very comfortable chairs, I could see that she was kind.

'Hey, Sister – what about coffee? This is Dr Delaney, who's going to work with Dr Sanders.'

'Going to work with Dr Sanders? Oh, my God!' Sister Eccles's face contorted like an elderly clown's. She wore two bright patches of rouge on her cheekbones which, together with her improbably dyed auburn hair, gave her defences against the ravages of Time a half ridiculous, half courageous look. She quickly turned to Harriet. 'I've just remembered,

Doctor. There's a lady in the dormitory who vomited during the night and I wonder if you could have a look at her, mmm?' She made a sort of sucking-whistling sound, with which I would soon become familiar. 'Lovely dress ... very ... very—' she sort of pranced around Harriet, of whom she was obviously fond, and then brought out the word triumphantly – 'Bohemian.'

Harriet closed one sea-green eye at me and went into the dormitory while Sister lurched off to get the coffee.

She came back with two cups on a tray. In the office she watched me sip mine, and then gave me a gentle but very thorough interrogation. I tried to follow suit and quiz her about Dr Sanders, but all she did was close her eyes, groan and say, 'Oh, my God, Dr Sanders ... Wonderful woman ... Works all the hours God sends her ... Mmmmmmm.'

The mention of her obviously electrified Sister Eccles, but then she switched to Harriet and went into eulogies of praise about her too.

'When I seen her first I thought, Oh, my God ... Mmmmm.' She did her little dance, flinging up her hands to her face like a Victorian heroine whose modesty had been outraged. 'The way she dresses ... and the voice ... I don't mean to be rude ... always an admirer of the medical profession, BUT ...'

After emitting her semi-snorting sound Sister Eccles went on to say that when you got to know her Dr Bentley was a 'lovely' little doctor, though 'easily hurt ... on her own', whereupon Harriet rushed in, and Sister skipped around her and rushed out.

'Nothing the matter with the old dear,' Harriet explained as she sat down and crossed her spectacular legs. 'She lost her teeth last night and probably bolted her supper. What do you make of Eccles?'

Before I could answer she threw her hands over her face and went 'Mmmm', doing such an expert imitation of Sister that I burst out laughing.

'She's sweet though, Eccles,' Harriet said. 'Very good with the patients. ...'

'She said the same about you,' I answered.

That didn't mean much, Harriet said. You got the greatest

admiration from Eccles if you called at regular intervals, didn't frighten her and listened to her woes and those of her family.

As she smoked several cigarettes, Harriet told me that she was a Senior Registrar and that she had been at Bushy Park eighteen months. She was doing an MD thesis, and was trying to make up her mind whether to get married or go all out for a consultant's post. The decision was difficult because she wanted a large family, and she couldn't neglect her children and leave herself at the behest of a Regional Board's training scheme for Senior Registrars.

'I was an orphan meself,' she said, 'brought up by me Gran. So I want a clatter of children when I get married. Can't leave it too long because me pelvis is so narrow.' She sprang up and outlined her narrow hips with two small hands.

'Yeah, I'll have to make up me mind soon. You'd like Tom. He's a GP . . . very bright. I couldn't marry a dumbo 'cause the kids mightn't have brains.'

She sat down again and began to comb her hair. I couldn't help noticing that the comb was full of blond hairs and I thought that her fiancé must be fair till she looked at it herself and exclaimed, 'Jesus, that bugger Francis must have borrowed me comb last night.'

The notion that 'Francis' might be a woman was dispelled when she told me that he was a demonstrator in the University and was recovering from a breakdown.

'Swallows tablets by the gallon. I had all about his demented mother-in-law and his cancer phobia. Where the hell do I collect them? Listen . . .'

But then she looked at my hand and to my astonishment I found myself telling her that I was separated from my husband and had a teenage son. Usually I became mute if I tried to explain my unorthodox situation, but although Harriet's appearance and nasal accent took some getting used to, I understood why Sister liked her. Behind the gipsy look and the fashionably eccentric clothes, I sensed a perception that was unusual in a young doctor. Besides, outspoken myself, I enjoyed her forthrightness.

'Yeah, you've had a rough time,' she said. 'Of course, once

13

you have a child you're buggered. I'm on the Pill meself. Which reminds me—' She pulled out a silver holder, opened it and popped a pill into her mouth. 'I think this brand is making me a bit depressed; I'm going to have to change to something else.'

'Have you a headache, Doctor?' Sister had appeared momentarily in the doorway.

'No, wrong end, Sister,' Harriet said, and for an awful moment I thought she was going to explain what she meant.

After Sister had flitted onwards Harriet asked me conspiratorially if I'd met Dr Sanders.

No, I said, but I was wondering what she was like.

Well, said Harriet, Dr Sanders was like those intrepid women who walked through Arabia on their own and then wrote a book about it, or who sailed up the Amazon to collect botanical specimens. 'Indestructible, that's the word for her. She's got a vile temper. Her psychiatry's more suited to the bush, but give her her due, she works. Mark you, she thinks I'm a common slut, though I can't say I mind, I'm used to it. But you want to watch it on ECT mornings,' Harriet added, getting up.

'Why?' I asked.

Harriet laughed.

'Because Rose Sanders has a little habit of *throwing* things if she can't get into a vein. Well, tatty-bye, I'm off.'

CHAPTER TWO

Although years of working in mental hospitals had left me with a degree of toughness and toleration in dealing with eccentric colleagues, I must say that I dreaded meeting Dr Sanders more than ever after I had visited her ward.

In the sudden rush to get on the bandwagon of modernity, Bushy Park Hospital had renamed most of its wards after former Medical Superintendents, dropping the bleak system of numbering which represented the old custodial-care days. It wasn't so bad, Harriet explained to me later that morning, if

14

the Superintendent had a reasonable name, but some wards were called things like 'Tickle' and 'Winterbottom'.

'That's Jasper Ward, a ward for new admissions. Rosie does it, so I won't take you up there,' Harriet said, as we passed a passage. 'Doctor Jasper was one of the very early Superintendents. There's a picture of him in one of the rooms near the front. He had only one eye and suffered from insomnia. Nasty old bugger ...'

That afternoon, after a lunch during which I met a few of the other doctors on the staff, I made my way to Jasper Ward. There was a Sister sitting at her desk in the office, talking to a young male nurse in a short white coat. His hair was long and he looked nervous. When Sister, a middle-aged woman with nondescript features and thick horn-rimmed glasses, got up, the male nurse went out after giving me a rather hunted look.

I explained who I was and Sister crushed out the cigarette she'd been smoking. Would I like a cup of tea? As her glance had been wary, and because it was easier, I said 'Yes' and she went out of the room for a minute.

When she got back she was followed by a maid bearing tea on a tray.

'I'm Sister Pinner.' She passed me a scalding cup of tea and shovelled sugar into her own cup.

'I believe Dr Sanders is at a clinic?' I wanted to take soundings as to whether Rose Sanders knew I was working with her.

'Oh, yes,' Sister said, 'Doctor's always out on Monday and Tuesday afternoons. Have you met her?'

I said 'No' and Sister went on, 'Well, once you've got used to her, you'll find that she is very kind. Very kind indeed. And most conscientious in her work. Of course—' she paused and looked at me – 'Dr Sanders is Getting On. She has her own ways of doing things. I mean, she puts each new patient on her special kind of treatment.'

What did that consist of? I asked.

Well, Sister explained, the 'Number One Treatment' was bed, twice-weekly enemas and vitamins; 'Number Two Treatment' was enemas and vitamins and massive doses of fluids; and 'Number Three Treatment' was a once-weekly enema and daily vitamins. I could see what Harriet meant about bush psychiatry.

The ward held seventy patients, Sister went on, as we walked up to a very pleasantly furnished day room. There was a dressmaking class in progress at one end of it, and, at the other, a young nurse was helping some patients on with their coats before taking them on a walk.

Just then a young nurse, pink-faced and panting, appeared from behind us and told Sister that the new patient had arrived.

'She looks very old, Sister – and she's blind and deaf.'

'What?'

'Blind and deaf, Sister.' The young nurse looked apprehensive, as well she might since as we walked back down the ward Sister seemed to grow several inches in stature and her voice got several decibels louder. Outside the office stood a cluster of people around a wheelchair, in which was crouched a very old woman.

The Mental Welfare Officer, a Mr Keating, whose job it was to keep an eye on patients when discharged and bring them into hospital when they needed admission, seemed to view Sister with the same apprehension as the nurse. I was sorry for him because he was very young and ugly, and his clothes were shabby.

She didn't know *what* Dr Sanders would say, Sister declared, trying to stop the old woman in the wheelchair from climbing out of it. They had been told to expect a rather elderly patient who would be able to look after herself, but this patient was obviously past seventy and . . .

There was an ominous trickle and a pool of urine appeared at the side of the chair.

'. . . and incontinent, too.' Sister stared at the urine and then directed a nurse to mop it up. Where did Mr Keating think they were going to get the staff? Didn't he know that Jasper Ward wasn't geriatric and that they'd have complaints from other patients?

With visible effort Mr Keating jerked himself out of his timidity and said that it was Dr Carton who had arranged the admission, that it was a matter of urgency to get old Mrs Best into hospital, as the daughter who looked after her had had a heart attack, and that the patient was living in a ramshackle condemned house anyway.

'Well, nothing to be done then.' Sister seemed to accept the admission as inevitable and two young nurses began to wheel the patient up to the ward. 'But I don't know what Dr Sanders will say. Dr Carton is *always* sending us difficult patients. Last week it was a mentally defective girl who set fire to the curtains, and the week before it was that woman who broke three beds.'

'Mrs Best's things . . .' Keating handed Sister a battered bag, which she took into the office, allowing him to beat a diplomatic retreat.

'Nothing to be done with these, really, except burn them,' she said, as we stared at Mrs Best's pathetic bundle of belongings. There was a tatty old fur cape, a bundle of yellow vests and bodices that wouldn't fit a ten-year-old child, and two nightgowns that were grey and greasy. The smell from the clothes was sickening. 'I hope she hasn't got lice. The last old woman that was sent in was covered with scabies.'

When I was told that Mrs Best was ready for examination, I found that the nurses had given her a good bath and tied her damp white hair back with a ribbon.

Although Sister Pinner had put up what I thought was almost a cruel resistance to having the old woman, I noticed that her attitude to her was gentle and kind.

'Let's be having you, love.'

She managed to calm the old woman, who was bobbing about in the bed, flailing her scrawny old arms like a boxing kangaroo.

It was only with great difficulty that I was able to do a cursory examination because poor Mrs Best was so agitated that she slithered about to avoid being touched. As she was nearly eighty and obviously hadn't been eating properly, she couldn't understand why she had been moved from her familiar surroundings to a strange and terrifying place, where strong arms plunged her into a bath she didn't want, and made her lie still while someone with a rustling coat placed a cold stethoscope on her thin body.

Sister pulled the bedclothes up and asked the nurses to bring a cup of tea and some thin bread and butter.

'She's probably been living on cornflakes and toast,' Sister said as we walked away. 'She'll be much better after she gets fluids and vitamins. Well, we'll be seeing you again in the morning then, Doctor?'

I went away trying not to think about the following day. I was beginning to experience the well-remembered swirling in my stomach which came when explosions were due.

I was up on the ward at half past nine the following morning and I read in the report book that Mrs Best had slept well after the mild tranquillizer I had ordered.

'Good morning, Doctor.' Sister came into the office, followed by the young male nurse. He might look weak and willowy but I had noticed him sitting down and writing messages for a patient with bad sight, after which he helped another with a tremor to hold her cup of tea.

'I hear Dr Sanders.' Sister jerked her head at the male nurse, who slid out. As the heavy tread approached, Sister whispered that although the Matron had decided on integrating staff and putting male nurses on female wards, and vice versa, Dr Sanders didn't 'hold' with the system and said that she wasn't having a male nurse near *her* patients. So they were having to hide the male nurse until Dr Sanders got used to him, which, Sister was sure, she would in time.

'Where's that new woman who's supposed to be working with me?'

There was a crash as the door of the office was flung open and then Dr Sanders stumped in. She was in her sixties, not so much fat as broad, and her mass of flaming red hair would have been pretty if she had not screwed it on top of her head in such a tight bun that her rather protuberant eyes looked permanently surprised. She didn't wear a white coat and her baggy tweed suit looked as if she'd slept in it.

Sister introduced us and Dr Sanders muttered something I couldn't understand as we shook hands.

'Right – well, let's get to work. Now, what's been happening, Sister?'

She settled herself down at the desk and rammed a pair of spectacles on her nose. As her nose was very small, and the glasses were very large, she looked rather like a surprised owl.

Inspecting the ceiling, Sister said that they'd had an admission. 'An elderly woman, Dr Sanders.'

'What age?' Sanders made a noise like a minor volcano about to erupt.

'Over eighty . . . and she's blind and deaf. Needs a great deal of attention.'

'Dear God . . .' Sanders groaned. 'Was it Dr Carton again?'

'He sent her in, Doctor.'

Weren't they supposed to be running an admission ward? There were no geriatric beds in the rest of the hospital where Mrs Best could be sent when she got better, and no relatives who seemed fit to look after her. Hadn't they three seventy-year-olds already in the ward who seemed to be developing into long-stay patients?

Sister nodded her head in all the right places and Dr Sanders's face changed from baby-pink to claret red. She picked up the phone as if it were a hand grenade and asked to speak to Dr Carton, brushing aside the operator who must have said that Dr Carton was engaged.

'I don't care if he's seeing relatives. Tell him Dr Sanders wants a word with him.'

She kept up a flow of muttered curses until Dr Carton came to the phone.

'Is that you, Richard? I must say I think it's absolutely disgraceful of you to send us a patient like Mrs Best. I knew she was coming? I beg your pardon, but you told me you were sending an *elderly, ambulant* woman. This patient is old and ill, with no hearing or eyesight. You know damn well we're short-staffed up here and that this is our last vacancy. I *know* the other doctors do it but you're the *worst* offender. That defective girl you sent last week is *pregnant*, by the way – another little matter you didn't tell us about. What do you mean, conditions in Mrs Best's house? I don't *care* if she was giving her food to the cats and if she spat through the letter-box at you. I hope to God she got a bull's eye.'

She crashed down the phone and leaped to her feet in one

19

movement, and Sister and I followed her broad figure as she strode through the ward, brushing patients aside like a human fly-swat.

Like Sister's Jekyll-and-Hyde act, Dr Sanders's attitude changed when she saw old Mrs Best. She sat down on the edge of the bed and tried to talk to her, but the patient grabbed a fistful of red hair and had to be held by a nurse. So Dr Sanders ordered the Number Three Treatment, and we all went back to the office.

'Eunice Radley wants to see you next, Doctor,' Sister said.

'Did she go out on weekend leave with her mother?'

'Yes, you said she could go for the weekend. The thing is that she went out with her boyfriend . . .'

'That greasy-looking dago who has a police record?'

'Yes. The thing is that Eunice has told us this morning that she thinks she's pregnant.'

'Oh, God . . . after that other girl. As if we haven't enough to do. Bring her in.'

Things were going to Hell, Rose Sanders went on, while Sister went for the patient. Sometimes she wondered if she was running a ward or a knocking-shop. Many of the women and girls she saw seemed to be as promiscuous as cats. Of course, when they got pregnant it was only too easy to terminate.

The patient was a curvy blonde in a jumper that was shrunk in the right places and a skirt as big as a handkerchief.

'Morning, Doctor love.'

Sanders snarled that she was *not* to be called 'love', and why had Eunice gone out for leave after she, Dr Sanders, had said she wasn't fit?

'Dunno, Doctor lo . . . I mean, Doctor. I just felt fed up, shut in here like, and it was Billy's birthday.'

'Is Billy your boyfriend?'

'Yeah, that's right. He wants to marry me when me divorce comes through.'

'It's not through yet, and you have four children in care, and you've to get yourself sorted out before you think of re-marriage. What's this about being pregnant?'

'Well, it's either that or an early change . . .'

'Don't be ridiculous. How could you be on the change when you're only twenty-seven?'

'It goes like that in our family. Me Mam was only twenty-six when she had her change. But I think I'm in the family way, Doctor.' Eunice spoke with the certainty of one who knows the signs of pregnancy only too well. 'I wish I'd persevered with the coil instead of having it whipped out after me sister asked me if it chimed when I walked.'

'Right. We'll have a pregnancy test done.' Dr Sanders wrote on a laboratory form.

'I don't know,' she grumbled when Eunice went out. 'Loops, coils, intra-uterine devices, do-it-yourself abortion kits. There's no sin left. I thought she looked pale, Sister, so put her on Number Three.'

After we had drunk the coffee that was brought in to us, I ventured to say that I had better do some of my other wards.

'Yes, all right.' Rose Sanders pawed for her glasses and looked at me. 'We have ECT in the morning. Up here, nine-thirty.'

Harriet had warned me about Rosie's Electro-Convulsive Therapy, and although I got used to her and her methods, I always dreaded the ECT mornings, which invariably were accompanied by some unfortunate nurse's sobbing fit, or by irate directions having to be sent to the Theatre providing the needles. The fact was that Rosie was very bad at giving injections because, in spite of her years of practice, she was, quite simply, ham-handed. Dr Hedley and the others had, according to Harriet, made strenuous efforts to stop her doing ECT, but Rosie had a strong sense of duty to her patients and to the doctors and nurses who worked with her, and since she decided it was the senior doctor's duty to be present at the ECT sessions, present she would be.

Her attempts to get into a vein were accompanied by exclamations and curses.

'Get out of the light, blast you!' she'd shout at some unfortunate who she imagined was in her way.

'God damn it, you're too STOUT!' she'd accuse some cowering patient.

'Terrible veins, terrible.' This was said whenever her repeated attempts to get in failed, and she had to ask Sister to plunge the arm in warm water. The last resort was always 'Bring the hot water bottles'. Many a morning went by while the patients sat surrounded by hot water bottles, waiting for the heat to bring up their veins into visible ropes.

It was all worse when Dr Sanders was dieting, Sister said. Evidently the fast at Ramadan was nothing to Rosie's periodic attempts to lose weight. At these times she existed solely on grapes and the whole hospital trembled at her approach. Because she so enjoyed her ordinary heavily starched meals, forgoing them made her exceptionally cross and irritable.

The first, and really the last, serious run-in that Rosie and I had was over food. I came up to the Doctors' Dining-room one lunchtime feeling very hungry: there was nothing left except a dish of sausages, and as the potatoes looked soapy and the soup cold, I speared four sausages and was about to return to my place when I felt a heavy hand on my shoulder.

'Do you realize that *others* are waiting for some sausages, Delaney?'

Rosie looked like a cook who had been at the cooking sherry, and Dr Hedley, Harriet and all the others at the table had an air of watchful expectancy. Ten years ago I would have blushed and slid the sausages back in grovelling apology, but I was approaching middle age, I was very hungry, and I was beginning to think that Viney was right about my having made a mistake in coming north.

'Listen, Rosie,' I said, 'we're not back in the Sixth Form and you're not the Captain of the Hockey Team.'

I thought her green eyes would come out of their sockets and her mouth opened like a goldfish gasping for air, but she only grinned and rang for more sausages. Rosie never bore any malice.

CHAPTER THREE

It took me ages to adjust to living in the north. The town nearest to the hospital was a noisy bustling place where people charged about purposefully to do their business, without wanting to dally over a cup of tea. The shops had windows crammed full of clothes, which were of quite good quality, but as there was no effort made to make the windows look pleasant the effect was very off-putting. The colours chosen were pretty awful, too, and there was a specially ghastly shade of piercing pink which was a great favourite with the Haxton ladies. I called it 'Haxton Pink'. If you felt depressed and you went into Haxton and looked at the Haxtonians stumping along in their pixie hoods and macs, you could understand a little of what Eliot meant when he wrote 'The Waste Land'.

I wasn't helped very much by Harriet's sighs and groans about the lack of stimulation at Bushy Park. The other Senior Registrar was a huge Indian doctor called Dr Singh, who spent most of his time either going off on study courses or else talking about the ones he'd been on. Although he was always very pleasant and had the rather endearing charm of a carpet dealer who's trying to make you buy one of his wares, Singh was far too earnest to be amusing, and was so terrified about offending anyone that, Harriet reckoned, 'he'd grin if you told him you had cancer'.

'I can't understand why you left the Osbourne,' Harriet said to me six weeks after I'd arrived at Bushy Park. 'The consultants were much better there, and after all you were nearer London. You've come to a real Dullsville. And for what? It's not as if you're getting *taught* anything. There's only Roger Ashe who's really bright, and he's a stinker.'

She was giving voice to a nagging doubt that was getting bigger and bigger inside me. Why *had* I come north? The extra money wasn't as much as I'd worked it out to be, and Harriet was right when she said that I wasn't getting tuition. The other doctors at Bushy Park were friendly and decent, but as far as modern psychiatry went they weren't very interested in keeping up with new ideas.

Harriet was ambivalent about Roger Ashe. She admired his cleverness and the fact that he was the only doctor at Bushy Park with an MD, but his snobbishness annoyed her. Once, she told me, when she was talking to him in the hospital corridor she had felt her pants slipping and had made no effort to save them, just so she could see the expression on his face when they landed at his feet.

'Red briefs – and with a pin in them, too,' she added with satisfaction. '*That* was something to tell his wife!'

She was so perceptive that she could judge to a nicety how much anybody liked or disliked her, and she knew very well that she annoyed Ashe as much as she did Rosie, but for rather a different reason. Rosie disliked the girl's, to her, un-professional ways, and Ashe recoiled in horror at her plebeian accent and outspokenness. The other doctors regarded Harriet with a kind of fascinated affection.

I had met Ashe on two occasions: he was a cadaverous man who looked older than his fifty years due to his bald head and pallid skin. Because he suffered from bad bronchitis, he was often away on sick leave. It was said that the only reason he'd taken a job at a provincial hospital was because his wife's relatives wanted her near them, and this was important be-cause Mrs Ashe's father was a very rich beer baron.

While people put up with Rosie's rages because of her very evident goodness and generosity, Ashe was treated with re-spect because of his withering tongue, but his sarcasm and apparent coldness made everyone wonder uncomfortably just what he thought about them and, worse, what he said about them when they weren't there.

'And as for a *social* life . . .' I had to agree with Harriet there. Only someone like Lowry could find Haxton beautiful, and if you didn't like Beer and Bingo, you could find little else in the town that would stimulate you.

I didn't mind this, really. After the years of galloping around with newly qualified energy, I had now settled for a life in which there only seemed room for my work and looking after my son. Maybe it was still a subconscious wish that I must punish myself for the mess of my marriage and the years I'd taken to accept the fact that I was really a doctor, and not some creature who had passed her exam by a miracle and been conferred with a medical degree by some oversight. Whatever the reason, I seldom went out except to sneak off to the cinema on my own, or to change my books at the local library. There seemed to be nothing more important than to escape getting into trouble in my work and thus prevent the bank manager sending me censorious letters.

The thing that I'd watched in other doctors and swore would never happen to me, *could* never happen to me, was coming to pass: I was becoming too involved in my work. My life outside the hospital, apart from the time I spent with my son, was becoming less real and important than the time I spent with the patients. This meant that I was able to become far more confident and interested in my work but a bit of a bore socially, because I often wanted to talk about patients and that meant I felt happier in the company of other doctors. Not that I found them any more intelligent than others but because they *understood* what I was talking about and I didn't have to stop and explain.

I had been looking forward to starting out-patients' clinics again. My interest in out-patient work, where patients are referred by their own General Practitioner for a psychiatric opinion to a clinic which is usually held twice weekly at their own neighbourhood hospital, appealed to me in the same way that dances did when I was younger: you never knew what was going to happen next. Every time the door opened and a new patient walked in, there was a private excitement, and even when the patient *wasn't* new and had what was sometimes a boring catalogue of complaints and a psyche that wasn't really interesting, there was a satisfaction if you were able to keep that patient out of hospital and in the community.

Dr Ashe did a genteel clinic at Roxall Hospital, which was so small that he really didn't need any assistance. Dr Hedley had Singh to assist him, and Harriet attended the clinics of Dr Toby Mason, who was a fattish man of very limited cerebral attainments. He had a ruddy face, prematurely grey hair which made him look falsely academic, and a Scots accent which, together with his Edinburgh degree, made him appear sound and respectable at interviews. He was far too normal to appeal to Harriet, who puzzled him by her wild habits and patronized him by her undoubted cleverness.

'So there don't seem to be any clinics going at the moment,' Harriet announced one evening when she had asked me over to her house. My son was away at school, and due to a dirty fog we had all been more or less isolated in the hospital for almost three days. Even the ambulance drivers didn't venture through the murky pall, except to rumble up three times with patients who were so mentally ill that they constituted real emergencies. 'It looks as if you'll do Rosie's clinic when she goes on holiday. That's the real accolade of approval from Rosie – if she allows you to do her clinic.'

It was true that Rosie and I were working well together. After the sausage episode she had never really tried to bully me again, and although she still got into furies, especially on ECT mornings, the rages were never directed at me.

'Just as her treatments are based on The Bowel, her clinic is based on The Change,' Harriet went on. 'I think it was Ashe, yes, it must have been dear Roger, who made up the phrase "the Haxton Flush". Here, have another cup of coffee.'

Harriet's house wasn't just untidy: it was dirty. She'd had a party the previous night, and as her help hadn't turned up the room was stuffy with stale cigarette smoke, and I could see several beer-stains on the shabby carpet. There were three plates of half-eaten sausage rolls on the sideboard, and I could see that somebody had left a cigarette burning on the table. I knew that Harriet's offer of coffee didn't mean that she'd make one for me; she would if I asked her, but she really expected me to go into her tiny kitchen and make my own.

It was best to avert the eyes as much as possible in Harriet's kitchen. She ate mostly out of tins, and when she'd finished with them she flung them into her bin, often with a bad aim, so that they accumulated in a pile at the bottom of the sink. Once, I had called to find her reading a textbook and eating a tin of cold baked beans. She looked surprised when I stared at the tin, because she really wasn't very interested in food or drink. I often saw her absent-mindedly drink quite a lot, and there was absolutely no change in her.

When I got back to the sitting-room I found her staring into the mirror above the fireplace, and I knew what the next question would be: Did I notice any new wrinkles on her face? And then she would part her hair and look for any streaks of grey. Harriet had a phobia about growing old. There was only one thing she was sure of and that was her physical attractiveness.

Her early upbringing had made her unsure of her social and intellectual status, but she could always prove that she was desirable and this, as I explained to Rose when she grumbled that she didn't mind so much about Harriet's nymphomania as long as she didn't *speak* about her orgasms, was at the bottom of Harriet's attitude to men. To her, they were bedworthy or they were not; and if they were, she went to bed with them, first seducing them with a single-mindedness that should have been offensive but somehow wasn't. She didn't want to break up marriages, Harriet told me, and this I believed.

Sexual intercourse was Harriet's passport into reality, the necessary proof that she was alive, and better, still attractive. There was an oddly pathetic and Ophelia-like quality in Harriet's sexuality, and in spite of her habit of boasting about the prowess of the men she went out with and her own response, I often thought that the word 'nymphomania', which she tossed around about herself, really meant that she used sex to console herself, like a small child reaching for a sweet or sucking her thumb.

I wondered what Tom Riley's attitude to Harriet's *affaires* was. Harriet's fiancé was a big fair man who seldom spoke but at least, as Rosie said, was a doctor and didn't eat his peas with his knife. We both agreed that if he was as bright as Harriet said, he concealed it very skilfully. Fat and torpid, he sat massively on the outskirts of every discussion and only came to life when the food was brought in. Perhaps his skill in cooking made up for his intellectual discrepancies, Rosie said. Harriet couldn't cook at all, or rather, had never felt the necessity of learning to do more than make tea or boil an egg, but Tom was able to work wonders in the culinary department, even in Harriet's tiny kitchen.

'You look much younger than you are ... about twenty-four,' I told Harriet. It was true and it pleased her. In spite of her rackety life, the queer diet and the late hours, her skin was unlined, with the dewy look you get in children, and the whites of her eyes were very clear.

'It's not vanity, you know, the way I dread age.'

I knew that: her looks were really all that the girl was sure of, and when they went she couldn't envisage how she would tackle life. The great bribe that she used to make people (men, anyway) like her would be gone.

When I first met her, she told me sometimes she got depressed, and I had thought that this was really her sense of drama, which was acute, and a certain amount of self-pity, but as I got to know her I came to see that she got genuinely melancholic.

'I'll never make old bones' was a favourite phrase of hers, and whenever I allowed myself to think about her future, I agreed with her. There are a few people you meet who you realize have a doomed quality about them, and Harriet was one of them. I could see her in my mind's eye committing suicide when life became unbearable. I think she knew this herself, and once she told me that she'd like to spend the rest of her life safely tucked up in a small room in some quiet hospital.

'There's me MD thesis.' She scrabbled under a chair and threw a heap of papers at me, while she went out to make her own coffee.

I began to read. Anybody who doubted if Harriet had brains was in trouble: she was very bright indeed and as I read, or tried to read, what she had written about certain aspects of the biochemistry of schizophrenia, I was half amazed that such wide reading and lucidity of expression were present in the brain of a girl who could sit in a house that was like a tip, and half admiring at her skill in statistics and her familiarity with the new work done in the biochemical field.

'It's really very good, Harriet.'

'Yeah, I know. I'll hand it in soon. The Prof has approved it. Then I'll have to make me mind up about getting married. Whatever happens, I'm going to bomb out of this dump. I'm getting very depressed.'

She shot to her feet and went to the window. The whirling fog looked like thick, encroaching waves. I watched her pull the curtains and curse when one of them stuck. She came back to the fire and curled in a ball in front of it, shivering like an alley cat that has slithered in from some wild sortie.

I had enough Celtic respect for death to wonder about

Harriet's attitude to it. As she sighed and stared into the fire, I said, 'Are you afraid of death, Harriet?'

She shook her hair back and looked at me.

'No,' she said, 'I'm afraid of life.'

CHAPTER FOUR

I had thought that Ceri Thomas, the woman psychiatrist for whom I had worked in my first job, had been direct with patients, but Rosie dived into the most intimate matters with a confidence that cut out any embarrassment in either doctor or patient, and made me believe the many stories about her Flaming Youth, when she had been the only woman in an Army Mess. Indeed, when she was in the mood, Rosie herself liked to reminisce in a bawdy enough way, about such topics as the right time to leave a party, which was a delicate matter to judge because, according to Rosie, you had to stay long enough not to make the men feel that you were really a spinster in your soul, and yet not long enough for you to have to put up a vulgar fight for your virtue.

The years at the Osbourne had made me immune to conversation which was so blue at times that you felt there ought to be smoke, but I was still lacking in Rosie's confidence in dealing with sexual topics at out-patient level, and I thought this must be due to my very inhibited childhood and convent upbringing.

We certainly weren't given any help in taking a patient's history when we were medical students, mainly because sex in Ireland was still taboo. You would have thought that when we were doing gynaecology we would have been told something about the Change of Life and Frigidity, but not a bit of it. Probably because the textbooks were written by men, I never could find more than some very short paragraphs on the menopause, a phase which, according to Rosie, was responsible for many of the ailments that beset a woman between the ages of twenty-eight and fifty-eight.

We had to pass written and practical examinations in

gynaecology. I never liked the subject, and I used to think that the women patients who attended the gynaecological clinics were treated with a terrible lack of respect for their age and sex. They were mostly from the Dublin slums, and they would arrive at the clinic carrying bulging shopping-bags and accompanied by the roaring products of their lack of contraceptive knowledge. Having a child annually, and their habit of not going to the dentist when their teeth fell out, made many of them look years older than they actually were. The poverty, which was savage, meant that they couldn't afford to have anything done to their hair, other than sticking it into curlers like pipe-cleaners, which only made a wild-looking frizz. I remember delivering a baby to a poor mother living in a back-street slum and finding that there were no clothes for the infant; we had to use a newspaper for it while one of us cycled back to the hospital for some baby clothes.

When I think of what those unfortunate women put up with, I cringe a little, even today. When they arrived at the hospital to attend the clinic they were told to take off their underclothes and then to take their places on the assembly line for an 'Internal'. Uncomplaining, about ten women would hop up on narrow beds, presenting their lower regions for examination, their tops hidden by green curtains. A nurse gave the doctor their history, to which he would refer without bothering to move the curtain. Often, he used the nurse to get more facts, and she used to hop behind the curtain to elicit more information from the patient, who never seemed to think it 'off' that she seldom saw the doctor directly. Indeed, such was the reticence and guilt about sexual topics that the patient was often glad that she hadn't to face him.

A typical history might be taken something like this: the doctor, more often than not with an entourage of medical students, would start at the top of the curtained line of women – whose lower parts always seemed to me to be far more undignified-looking with their legs lifted up on stirrups than if they were completely naked and exposed – and proceed down the line, after which another group of women would replace the first contingent.

'Mrs Flynn complains of "something coming down" and passing water when she coughs or laughs.'

Many of the women, due to constant child-bearing, suffered from a 'prolapse', in which the womb or uterus sinks down due to lack of support, and causes a host of annoying symptoms.

'How many children, Missus?' The nurse peeped behind the curtain, and a ripe Dublin voice answered, 'Five, and four mistakes.'

'Mistakes' was Dublinese for a miscarriage.

'And what are you complaining of, Mrs Flynn?'

'I feel a "drawing" when I passes me water, and last week when I had the flu, I wet the bed every time I coughed. Indeed, I have to go round wearing a bit of a towel.'

'Yes, yes.' The gynaecologist always seemed to be afraid that some lack of the proper reticence would make the patient offend against Holy Modesty. 'Now relax, Mrs Flynn, I'm going to examine you.'

'All right, Doctor.' Mrs Flynn was so used to having babies that the internal examination was as nothing.

I had been shown how to feel the womb. I had studied the diagrams in the textbook which showed it neatly tucked behind the bladder. I had learned its position off by heart, 'anteverted' and 'anteflexed', and I had been shown the correct way to palpate it, with one gloved hand in the vagina and one pressed gently over the lower abdomen, but I could never feel the womb with any certainty in a patient.

We used to attend the gynaecology clinics given by a thin, granite-faced man, who it was said owed his hospital position to being related to someone high up in the Government. He had little humour and was a fanatical Catholic, and I think he offered up his teaching in atonement for his sins, because he really had a great deal of patience in dealing with us students.

One afternoon I had tried to feel the womb on four women, without success, and I was beginning to wonder whether the organ existed, although to give me my due, one of the patients was sixteen stone and another was so tight that when I put my hand in, I could hardly get it out.

31

'Well, Miss Delaney, have you felt the uterus?'

The gynaecologist loomed behind me as I passed on to a new patient.

I began to do a vaginal examination and made the proper movements that were supposed to make uterine examination easy. I decided to lie and I said confidently, 'Yes. Yes, I can feel the uterus.'

The gynaecologist gave a wintry smile.

'Miss Delaney says she can feel the uterus in this patient, which is extraordinary because—' he beckoned to the nurse – 'I believe the patient had a hysterectomy, which all of you doctors will know means removal of the womb, ten years ago ...'

The nurse popped her head around the screen. 'Did you, Missus?'

'I did indeed, Nurse. That darling doctor in front done it after me last was born. John Joe, his name is, and he was ten pounds when he was born, a big bullister of a boy, and I dunno what damage he did me for I was advised to have Everything Out ...'

My foundations of knowledge for doing Rosie's clinic were, therefore, very shaky; so I decided to go and see Dr Molyneux, an acromegalic lady who was the consultant gynaecologist to the Haxton hospitals. She did a stately clinic at Bushy Park twice a week.

What was her treatment for the menopause? I asked her. In my young days I had been taught that women were supposed to battle through this difficult phase in their life. Rosie used a great deal of Piperazine, which she always referred to as 'The Pips', a drug that contained Vitamin C and had the property of causing flushing on its own, so that it was very difficult to know what was due to the drug or to the woman's own physiology. Perhaps there was some newer and more up-to-date treatment? But Dr Molyneux didn't believe in giving *any* drugs to women at their menopause. The only useful ones were, she thought, dangerous, and she would advise me not to give anything other than mild tranquillizers if the woman complained.

'There's far too much importance given to what is after all

a natural physiological process,' she added. 'If a woman *thinks* she's going to have a bad menopause, then she will: it's what some of your psychiatrists call "bad conditioning", to make a woman think that because she's reached a certain age, she'll suffer.'

I agreed with Dr Molyneux, but as Rosie's patients had been conditioned for years to think of their problems as meno-pausal, I wondered what on earth I was going to say to the patients to get their minds off what should be a natural pro-cess. It was going to be a difficult task, because Rosie believed so much in a glandular basis for middle-aged troubles that she extended her theory to fit males, and gave it as her opinion that men, too, had a menopause which could be nasty. It showed up in such behaviour as running off with the *au pair* or pinching young girls' bottoms.

I remembered Dave Hedley. He had done Rosie's clinic one week when she had reluctantly been forced to bed with flu, and to ward off a similar attack he had popped a Vitamin C tablet into his mouth during the clinic. A patient was going to town on the length and extent of her red flush when, to his dis-comfort, he felt the Vitamin C begin to suffuse his face with scarlet. To his even greater horror, he saw that the patient had noticed. She stared at him in fascination. 'By gum! Dr Sanders knows a thing or two! She *told* me men 'ad 'em, but I wouldn't have believed it till I seen yours, Doctor!'

CHAPTER FIVE

When I went down to take Rosie's clinic the following week, I was aware of the peering glances from the rows of women who were sitting outside the clinic-room door. Several were sewing or knitting, and a few had brought flasks of tea.

'Three ladies went home when they heard it wasn't Dr Sanders,' Sister told me as I took off my coat.

My efforts to tailor the clinic by lengthening the intervals between appointments failed. To a woman, Rosie's patients went on a sort of sit-down strike by saying that they'd forgotten what their GP looked like, and Dr Sanders had said they could come here as long as they liked. This was true. All the GPs off-loaded their time-consumers onto Rosie who was far too tender-hearted in fact to dream of sending back her patients. Some of the case notes were so old that they looked like maps of Treasure Island.

Beaten in my first ploy, I sat and listened for two hours to the patients' litanies of menopausal woes. One woman pulled sheafs of paper out of her bag, saying she only remembered things she wanted to tell the doctor on the bus going home. She thrust it into my hand, and I had to say I would take it back to the hospital and read it there.

Palpitations, 'Mazy do's' (a term much used to describe giddiness), insomnia, fits of temper, frigidity, the inevitable hot flushes ... By now I knew how much importance Rosie attached to the Hot Flush, so I didn't have to depend on reading her writing, which looked as if a drunken mouse had got into an ink bottle and scurried over the paper. The number and extent of the hot flushes was a great topic of conversation, and quite a few of the patients told me about the rival Cold Flush in which Dr Sanders was so interested. My understanding of these phenomena was limited by the fact that all the ladies were on the Pips, and were thus flushing long before they reached the change. Indeed, I sometimes had to appeal to youth in order to break the patients' menopausal conditioning. When I suggested to one attractive girl that surely it was very matronly to think that she should be approaching the change at thirty, she said, 'I don't think so, Doctor. Dr Sanders said that an Early Change was a sign of being highly strung, and I'm highly strung.' Whatever Rosie said was regarded as Holy Writ.

You couldn't get away from the fact that for many of her patients Rosie's clinic was the highlight of their week. Many were lonely, either because they were widowed or else had bored their relations to gibbering point. The young women were lonely because their husbands were doing overtime or studying: when they arrived home, they switched on TV or buried themselves behind newspapers, while their wives were bursting to tell them about the long cheerless day, unrelieved by relatives and friends calling because, as one young woman said, 'These days they're all out working.' To come into the clinic meant that you met other women with bigger and better symptoms than your own. You could spend a masochistically enjoyable time watching the patients going in and out of the other clinics that were held that afternoon at the hospital: if you were lucky, you caught a glimpse of a trussed figure on a trolley or heard the unnerving cry of a terrified child. It was all better than sitting at home, drinking solitary cups of tea and watching the soap operas on telly.

Rosie didn't mind children coming, either; indeed, she had her own brand of child psychiatry and was ever ready to leap into the difficult waters of Marriage Guidance, so the chatter of the women patients was always interposed with the noise of playing or impatient children. And when you did get to Rosie, she greeted you as if she was really pleased to see you, instead of looking huntedly at her watch, the way your own doctor did. And you could say anything to Dr Sanders . . .

'Dr Sanders said that me libido might increase – what does that mean, Doctor?' one rather prissy-looking patient asked. She fell into the category which Roger Ashe would describe uncharitably but accurately as 'Dull and Stupid', and she obviously thought that her libido was some organ near her liver. I cursed Rosie inwardly and tried to explain, but as my voice faltered the patient glared at me, gathered up her bag and said that she was sure Dr Sanders didn't mean *that*.

Foiled in my attempts at trimming Rosie's clinic, I gave up trying and simply carried out her function as a wailing wall. I told the patients to keep taking the Pips until Dr Sanders got back, and wrote out prescriptions for massive doses of vitamins.

Only one patient dared to question the treatment: she was a bright schoolmistress, who said she had read that Piperazine tablets were given to pigs to de-worm them, and she failed to see how de-worming in someone who hadn't got worms could help their nerves. This was a tricky one, as it is perfectly true that Piperazine is given to animals, so I had to pull myself quickly together and try to make sense out of Rosie's conviction that all nervous trouble was made worse by the accumulation of toxic products and that 'flushing out', as she called her Pips treatment, was very effective.

Ashe wandered into the dining-room the day after I had done the first clinic, and commented on my account of it.

'We can't ignore the fact that the patients feel much better after they see Rosie, but of course that's due to her ebullience and the projection of her own personality. As I told you, one can only be consoled by the thought that there are worse clinics in this ghastly area. I really can't understand why you came north, Dr Delaney. People are so *rude* up here, digging one in the ribs and mistaking lack of manners for courageous outspokenness.'

I listened to Roger Ashe telling me about the terrible time he had when he had done a short stint in general practice. The surgeries had been bad enough, but having to visit patients was infinitely worse.

'The sordidness of it,' he moaned. 'The smell of wet clothes in the hall and the dishes of rancid butter on the table. Once I even caught *fleas*.'

Listening to him, I wondered, as I had done on many occasions, why Ashe continued to work as a doctor when people and their smells upset him so. I had heard it said that he had to get out of the house periodically because Mrs Ashe was very bad-tempered.

'Of course, the *worst* clinic to have to do without a doubt is Madley clinic. Even the name is ridiculous. Dr Ellison, who does it at the moment, has had a coronary, so we watch his health with interest.'

I had met Henry Ellison, a small, very intense man, who was so overweight and smoked so much that it was no wonder he had heart trouble.

Madley, according to Ashe, was an industrial town some fifteen miles away, and the hospital was situated down near the canal. It always seemed to be raining there; the smell from a near-by knacker's yard permeated everything, and the people, if I could believe it, were more stupid and rude than the Haxton inhabitants.

'I did it once a week – I refused to go twice – when Ellison had his last "do", so I know. They're always threatening to

36

close the hospital; indeed, it looks so shaky I wonder it doesn't fall asunder, but they've never got round to it. Singh used to go and help Ellison last year but he got out of it, as these devious Orientals are very good at doing, by putting in for study leave. I'm afraid that if someone *is* needed to do the clinic, the newcomer is always given the task . . .'

It was a good thing that I was prepared for Madley. Two weeks later Hedley called me to his office and said that, since Dr Ellison had had a very bad heart attack, he'd have to ask me to cover his clinic at Madley for an indefinite period.

I was overcome by a feeling of paranoid rage. I hated covering other people's clinics for long periods. It was rather like fostering a child: you got the clinic shaped and running as you wanted it, and then the rightful owner turned up. And I wouldn't even be learning anything, if what Ashe said was true. With everybody's commiserations ringing in my ears, I decided to find Harriet.

She seemed to have been infused with tremendous energy during the previous two weeks. I often came across her writing in the case sheets and occasionally passed her racing along the corridors, hair streaming behind her like a banner, and brief skirt showing a flash of red petticoat (she never bothered with a white coat).

I'd tried ringing her in vain on four successive evenings before I finally got through. She sounded very cheerful; Tom was out that night and I could come over right away.

The house was as smelly and untidy as ever, but Harriet herself looked as if she was charged with electricity. Her eyes blazed, there were two patches of bright red on her cheeks, and she never stopped talking and smoking. She had nearly finished her MD thesis, she had put in for leave to attend a psychiatric meeting in London, she had received some back money from the income tax, and she had been on a buying spree. It was all a marked contrast to her depressed mood of a few weeks ago.

'What do you think, Joyce? Takes a few years off me?' She twirled around in a pair of culottes, enjoying the way they emphasized her small waist. 'We're going to a party tomorrow night and I'll wear this. I'm not going with Tom – don't tell him about it. No, you see, I met this bloke at the University last week. He's got the sexiest eyes – unstable, of course, but then all the best people are . . . I'll answer it!'

She snatched up the phone and I heard her advising the person on the other end on how to take heart tablets. Harriet always had troupes of friends and members of the nursing staff who involved her in their illnesses. She told me once that this involvement helped what she called her 'missionary zeal', but I think that some of it was due to her undoubted kindness and feeling for other people in trouble.

She crashed down the phone and lit a cigarette, then pulled a coat over her culottes and a picture hat over her long hair. I noticed that her hair was matted and uncombed, and when she came close to me I saw that she was sweating a lot and that her lips were dry and cracked. There was no tell-tale sign from her pupils that she was on drugs, but I knew enough about her to know that she wasn't herself. Her energy, speed of talk and flight of ideas made her seem manic.

'Are you eating, Harriet?' That was fairly inoffensive.

''Course I am. You know me. Bag of crisps and a sani.'

'Sani' was Scouse for sandwich, and it was true that she never ate much, but her clothes were looser on her, and, seeing me staring at the dark smudges under her eyes, she looked into the mirror and said, 'This bloody Pill isn't suiting me. I look terrible, don't I? And I'm not sleeping.'

She turned up the record player and did a little dance around the room, humming to herself. The phone went again and I heard her say that she'd be over to the hospital soon.

'Sorry, I'm on duty,' she said, lighting another cigarette from the butt of the first one. 'There's a patient with a temperature to be seen, and one of the nursing staff came on duty with a pain in his ribs. Oh, I must send these bloody people some money. They're threatening me with a solicitor. I owe them a hundred or two.'

'For clothes?' I asked, as she pulled out a bill and her cheque-book. I noticed that her bag was bulging with papers.

'Yeah, I bought a lot last week. Can't take it with you, Joyce. No pocket in a shroud, like the man said. Let them have a fiver. I needed some style to cheer me up, didn't I? And I feel much better than I did ... Too much energy now ... Where's the fags?' She seemed to have forgotten the cigarette burning on the mantelpiece.

I tried to keep my face deadpan, but I felt an ominous click in my mind and I knew that the quick change in her from depression to elation reminded me of the classic description of manic-depressive psychosis, a mental condition genetically transmitted and characterized by mood swings. I shook off my idea as quickly as it came, reminding myself that working in a mental hospital made me too quick to pigeon-hole people and diagnose. Manic-depressive psychosis was commoner in pyknic people, and Harriet was slender, and I didn't know whether there was any instability in her family. When I got home I found that I had forgotten to tell Harriet about the Madley clinic, but somehow even if I'd remembered, I had an idea that her attention was so fleeting at the moment that she wouldn't be much help.

Neither Rosie nor Ashe seemed to have noticed Harriet's heightened mood, and so I called at Rosie's room one evening soon after this, having been invited to a party the following Saturday at Harriet's. Fortunately I had the excuse that I was on duty, because I didn't want to go.

'Have you been asked to Harriet's party?' I watched Rosie throw a shoe at the cat that had leaped onto the mantelpiece.

'There *was* some sort of phone call from her.' Rosie was meant to be leaving in a few months to live in her small cottage in Wales and she was far more irritable than when she was fasting. Her thirty years of hospital work had made her as ill-prepared to face life outside as a contemplative nun. 'But she was talking so much rubbish that all I could make out was something about Saturday night. I simply said that if she'd looked at the notice board she'd have seen I was away for the weekend.'

'Do you think Harriet is well, Rosie? She looks tired.'

'No food, late hours and men ...'

'It's just that I feel a bit worried about her.'

Rosie grunted. When I was as old as she was I would recognize a psychopath when I saw one, because that's what

39

Harriet was, a tiresome little psychopath, and surely I had enough to worry me, with a son to bring up on my own, without wasting time on a freak like Harriet?

Rosie had decided not to like Harriet and that was that. Like myself, she could tell horrific stories of the days of the Grand Eccentrics in mental hospitals, but they had all of them been *gentlemen*. She deplored the entry into medicine of the Grant People, who took off their jackets to eat, spoke with their mouths full and used bad grammar. Filled as she was with professional pride, she hated Harriet's common touch and her familiarity with porters and nursing staff. Only the week before she had called me to the front hall and pointed out Harriet, who was perched on the porter's desk showing a great deal of leg and tossing back her hair.

'I heard the porter call her by her *first* name,' Rosie muttered.

There was no use in trying to say more to her. I would be a greater help to Harriet keeping my mouth shut. I would have to hope that while I was busy at Madley, Harriet's life would swing back on course again of its own accord.

CHAPTER SIX

The following week I drove over to Madley to do the clinic, and the dreariness of the drive, coupled with the slashing rain, fulfilled all Roger Ashe's gloomy prognostications. I had thought that Haxton's centre was unattractive until I saw Madley; there were a few big shops situated around the ugly-looking Town Hall, after which all effort at a shopping centre petered out and there were just rows and rows of dirty-looking shops. Five minutes before reaching the town, the smell of the knacker's yard assaulted my nostrils.

The hospital was situated at the bottom of a winding street, and I couldn't blame the Regional Board for intending to close the place within two years. It had been designed as a cottage hospital and held about sixty patients suffering from surgical and medical complaints. Whoever planned the building must have believed that hospitals should look cheerless and grim, because after your heart had sunk several feet at the sight of the squat grey front of the place, it dipped still further when you went inside and tried to make your way amongst the warren of small dark rooms.

The Out-Patients' was at the back of the hospital and the bare waiting-room reminded me of a poorhouse. There were no curtains, no pictures; the patients sat on uncomfortable bare benches. On the wall two notices depicted the lethal effects of smoking: one that drew the eye magnetically showed cigarettes assuming the shape of coffins.

The two secretaries who sat at their typewriters in the small room outside my office were pleasant enough. One of them followed me into the office and introduced herself as Mrs Sweetman. She apologized for the austerity of our surroundings. 'It's Matron, you see,' she explained. 'She ... well, she doesn't *understand* the Psychiatric Clinic.'

I was used to this sort of attitude in general hospitals, where the psychiatrist is still regarded at worst as a dangerous oddity who doesn't really work, and at best a luxury who doesn't have to be considered when there's money needed.

I stared out of the window, eyeing the outlines of a murky slag heap in the distance. The curtains were dirty, and the walls and ceiling could certainly have done with a wash. When I sat in the rickety chair behind the table I wobbled, and for one paralysing moment thought I was going to suffer the indignity of falling onto the dusty floor.

'I keep asking the carpenters about that hole in the floor ... I'm sorry, Doctor.' Mrs Sweetman rushed to my rescue.

No wonder James Ellison had had a coronary, I thought, as I leafed through the stack of case notes piled in front of me. It was as hard to get information about old patients from Ellison as it was from Rosie. Ellison didn't like writing notes at all so you had very little information to go on, and he had an infuriating habit of using the abbreviation 'ISQ' (In Status Quo). This didn't help because you had no real idea of what the patient was like in the first place. I had heard Ashe describe his difficulty in dealing with a big blonde patient, who had sat expectantly in front of him while Ashe stared down at what

Ellison had written about her under 'History'. There, showing up starkly on the white page, was one single word: 'Deprived'.

Mrs Sweetman came in looking pink and flustered. The first patient was new: her name was Victoria Condron and she had turned up last week only to find that there was no clinic. This week she was grumbling that she had had to wait twenty minutes.

'Very cheeky, Doctor.' Mrs Sweetman's kind middle-aged face looked red. 'She's giving us all the rounds of the kitchen sink. *And* she arrived in a taxi.' The last seemed really to dispose of Mrs Condron in her estimation.

The girl who came in projected her anger like an almost visible cloud. She didn't look at Mrs Sweetman, who crept out after giving me a long sympathetic look.

'I thought I'd see a man doctor!'

Mrs Condron crossed her legs aggressively. She was about twenty-five and would have been pretty in a rosy-cheeked, blue-eyed way if she hadn't looked so explosive. I tried to read the letter from the GP, after Mrs Condron had listened to my explanation about Dr Ellison with an air of one who has been deceived by many doctors in the past.

'This is a very difficult patient,' Dr Masters, the GP, had written. 'There is a long family history of neurosis (patient's grandmother died in a mental hospital) and Mrs Condron has complained of many physical symptoms for which no organic cause has been found. She has seen various specialists and will, I am sure, fill you in herself on her various ailments, as she is very articulate. Her husband and she do not get on very well and their little girl (who suffers from epilepsy) is attending a day nursery. I should be glad of your advice.'

'He's trying to offload me, Masters . . .'

I wasn't going to be manoeuvred into the all-too-easy situation of listening to a patient denigrate her doctor. At any rate, I'd been at Bushy Park long enough to know that for some odd and unexpected reason Madley had an excellent crowd of GPs. They knew their patients, sent polite letters and were well abreast of the new drugs on the market.

'I'll have to ask you a few questions, Mrs Condron,' I said.

She groaned dramatically. 'Questions, questions ... Listen, I've seen so many doctors and none of them seem to be able to cure me. All shunting me off to see another specialist. And now Masters thinks I'm a nut case ...'

She began to sob loudly and I had to try and force myself to remember that the first referral to a psychiatrist could be very traumatic, especially in a place like Madley where there was the danger of patients coming from the same neighbourhood.

'You haven't seen me before. Have a cigarette.'

'Fags are dangerous.'

I was ready for that one, which I fielded by saying that I was so well aware of that fact I had given up smoking myself, but that there *was* the odd occasion, such as now, when a cigarette might be permissible.

She blew her nose, pulled out a packet of cigarettes, lit one, after waving the packet at me, and then began to smoke with furious puffs.

What was the matter with her, I asked again.

'Dunno – that's for *you* to say. That's what makes me so twitched ... I don't feel normal.'

'Let's start at your childhood.'

'Oh, why do you want to go digging that far back? Can't you just give me something to make me feel better?'

I switched the light on. The rain was pattering against the murky window but the curtains were too skimpy to pull. My watch said that Mrs Condron had been in with me for over forty-five minutes.

'Listen, Mrs Condron,' I said, 'I can't decide what's wrong with you before knowing something about you.'

'I've *told* doctors the answers to all those questions before. Ask Masters ...'

'*Doctor* Masters ...'

'I didn't come up here to be made to feel like a kid who keeps saying the wrong thing.'

'And I have other patients to see outside.'

'You're going to throw me out. Good!'

Her tears had stopped and I could see that part of her was enjoying acting out the aggression that was eating her. I was feeling cramped and tired already and Mrs Condron seemed to typify the difficult patients that Ashe had said existed nowhere but in Madley. The idea of doing a clinic here for an indefinite period was terrible.

Mrs Condron jumped to her feet and, before I could even make a gesture of defence, gave me a stinging slap on the cheek. I was horrified at the temptation to give her stupid, tear-stained face a crack in return.

She stood looking down at her hand which was still out-stretched, and began to cry again.

'Don't you ever do that again.' I could feel my cheek going red, and all of a sudden Viney's face appeared before me, mouthing, 'I told you so.' Why hadn't I taken his advice and stayed in the civilized south?

'I'm sorry, Doctor. I didn't really mean it. You won't tell Ma ... Doctor Masters, will you? He's good, really ... He came out to see me at three in the morning last Saturday. I suppose I'd better go.'

I wanted her to go. I knew that there would be a very long haul before I could do anything for Mrs Condron, and that this would be only the beginning of many troublesome inter-views. But, still, to let her go would be a complete therapeutic failure for me, and poor Dr Masters would have no one to share the buck with. I forced myself to speak quietly.

'Let's forget this and start from the very beginning ...'

Damn, I sounded like Helen Keller, and I didn't *feel* like her in the least.

After another half-hour I managed to get some facts from Mrs Condron. She had had a childhood dominated by an un-stable mother, who brought her up in the shadow of her own unsatisfactory marriage, and now she had married unhappily and for the last three years had felt tired, lonely and depressed. Her husband had said that the reason their child had epilepsy was due to Mrs Condron's mother being mentally ill.

Once started, there was no stopping Mrs Condron and I had to tell her again that there were other patients waiting to see me. I asked her whether she could come back in two weeks' time and the tenuous communication we had established snapped quickly when she tried to bully me into seeing her the following week. She wouldn't accept my explanation that the lists were full due to the backlog occurring after Dr Ellison's illness, and, snatching up her bag, she glared at me, saying that she'd bet anything I had forged my appointments lists. She knew how doctors liked to pretend that they were always busy, and anyway she couldn't come in two weeks because her mother was coming. When I tried to say that I'd like them both to come, she announced that her mother only had to look at a hospital to bring on one of her 'turns'.

I could feel the ominous scratchy feeling of an impending cold starting at the back of my throat, and I wished that Victoria Condron would go and leave me in peace. I didn't think that I could really do much for her; there was far too much resistance in her, and anyway she was quite obviously going to cling to her symptoms so that she could manipulate things to suit her.

After the girl had swept out with a furious bang of the door, Mrs Sweetman came in sighing. Mrs Condron had gone in without an appointment and Miss Rivers, the Matron, was pale with rage after having had to tell Victoria twice to put out her cigarette.

'Do you want your tea first, or will you see the Tasker family?'

I said I would have my tea while I saw the patients. They were Father, a retired army RSM who was subject to minor fits; Mother, who was on the change; and son Ambrose, who had a tic and occasional sickness. The bulging pile of notes indicated that the Taskers were 'regulars' at the clinic and Mrs Sweetman pointed to a collection of typewritten letters at the back of the case notes. They were angry missives directed to various bodies such as the educational authorities and the Council, complaining about the injustices meted out to Mr Tasker and his family. From the style and use of words I could see that Mr Tasker was paranoid but intelligent, and I remembered Viney's axiom that the most difficult and dangerous patients were the bright ones who suffered from paranoia – all Hitlers in miniature, according to Viney.

The Tasker family's entrance entailed my getting up to pull out two more chairs and hold a fat sleeping infant while Mrs

Tasker, a portly woman in her forties, settled herself. The husband, a small waxen-faced man, directed the removal of his wife's and son's raincoats, and then took up a place sitting between them.

Anticipating a grumble, I said that I was sorry for the delay in seeing them.

'What do you think of this coat?' Mr Tasker held up his son's navy blue mac. 'Almost eight pounds!'

Poor Amby's small white face quivered with embarrassment and he stared down at his bony knees.

'Hand to mouth, that's how we exist, Doc. And does the Gover'ment care that I fought for me country? And the fact that I was struck down in me prime by a brain disorder? No, you needn't apologize for keeping us, Doc. We're used to it – aren't we, Annie? Two hours you waited at Doctor's surgery last week for your blood pills, didn't you?'

'That's right, Harold. Anyway, we seen that the young lady who was with you was very ill.'

'Yes,' agreed Harold, 'she seemed to me to be a product of the pressures facing young people today. See that baby, Doc?'

I stared at the child who had been deposited on the examining couch. It lay dead still, a fat white fist in its mouth.

The baby, explained Mr Tasker, belonged to a neighbouring couple, both of them students, and it was only with the few pounds a week given for the child's keep that the Tasker money was able to go round at all, even though Annie Tasker had a goitre and anaemia and really wasn't fit to cope with a child.

There was nothing written recently about the Taskers in Ellison's writing, and what little he *had* written seemed to indicate that the family had come in the first instance because of Ambrose getting his Eleven-Plus and then being unable to cope at the new grammar school. His parents had leaped on the Ellison wagon; he believed that you shouldn't treat patients in isolation but should see the whole family. From what I could make out, the family's once-monthly visit was so that they could report on their ailments and, most important of all, give Mr Tasker a chance to get rid of his excess rage.

46

I tried to head off Harold Tasker from discussing the reasons why Dr Ellison had had a coronary. I didn't have to tell him, Harold said; he had noticed for some time that Dr Ellison was getting very edgy.

'Used to rub his nose a lot, didn't he, Annie? And that throat-clearing . . .'

'Aye. 'Scuse me.' Annie lumbered to her feet; the baby had begun to cry in a thin wail. She stuck a dummy into its mouth and after giving a surprised snort the child went to sleep again.

Mrs Tasker glanced at her spouse, who was obviously the spokesman for the family, and then dug her elbow into her son's side.

'Stop picking your nose, Amby. Well, me husband's not so bad, Doctor, but I had flu since I seen the other doctor and it's left me proper weak.'

'Can't hardly cut a sausage,' Mr Tasker put in. 'And the baby's parents has their exams on. Terrible, it's been. Course, our Amby's not so bad 'cos he's settled down at that new school. If it wasn't for certain boys who seem to have a down on him he could really settle. I think that really upset me wife, Doctor. See, we've always surrounded Amby with love and affection and he's never met up with nastiness. Even if I could afford it I wouldn't have TV in me house, all them bed scenes. I tell you, in all me years in the Service I never heard such language as they put out in those plays. Any road, there's this crowd of foul-mouths who tried to corrupt Amby . . .'

Mr Tasker pointed at his son, who began to move his feet around restlessly, and then he winked at his wife, who leaned over to me, smelling of camphor and onions, and said rather loudly, 'Gave him pictures of naked women to look at.'

I made suitable noises of sympathy and Mr Tasker said he'd written what he called 'a strong letter' to the school's Head. There was going to be no chance of seeing Ambrose on his own, I knew. It was a wonder to me that the child was as stable as he appeared, suffocated as he was by his parents' own neuroses and their heavy concern for him.

I let Mr Tasker have his head in a long soliloquy about the harshness of Fate that had given him a brain but no education. He had noticed stupid men earn more money, and had watched in helpless fury as the less able outstripped him. There was no doubt that Life had dealt him a dirty hand, and I found myself beginning to admire his Quixote-ish tilting at bureaucratic and administrative windmills.

As the baby began to stir and the unmistakable smell of a wet nappy filled the room, Mr Tasker prompted his wife to tell me about the new lodger.

'We got this spare room, Doctor, and as me sister's eldest wanted lodgings I let him have it.'

'At a cheap rent,' Mr Tasker butted in. 'Anyway, Doctor, the wife has always been a good cook and kept the home nice, but there's no pleasing Cedric – that's the nephew's name. I don't know where he got all those ideas. Wants to stay in the bath for an hour at a time, listens to music full blast late at night and says Mrs Tasker's cooking isn't "seasoned" enough. I say it's putting on the wife, like, but she says that she owes it to her sister.'

'We'll give Cedric a chance.' Mrs Tasker slobbered softly over the baby. 'After all, me sister always said that he was different – sensitive like ...'

'Selfish, I'd say.' Mr Tasker looked martyred. 'But again, Doctor, beggars can't be choosers and the money's useful. Same time next month?'

I staggered out of the hospital at half-past six. The darkness covered Madley's ugliness in a merciful pall.

When I got to the hospital next morning, I met Harriet flying towards me, wrapped in a black cape and clutching a parcel.

'Look, Joyce, cookery books ... I'm really going to start learning how to cook.'

There were four expensive-looking volumes and a bill stuck on top.

Harriet's eyes were a blue-green glitter and the circles under them were larger than ever. She told me that she was on duty and had been on a ward to see a patient who had collapsed. She was now dashing home to wash herself, as she had just leapt from her bed to go on the call.

'Not that I was asleep. I wake every morning at five now

and smoke or drink coffee till it's time to get up. Hey, here's Dreamboat . . .'

Roger Ashe came through the door, loping along in elegant suede shoes, carrying a briefcase. The camelhair coat would have looked pretentious on anyone else.

'Hi, Rog, how's your love-life?' Harriet shrieked raucously as she raced off.

As he considered the disappearing figure he shuddered. 'Really, that girl should be put down.' He turned to me. 'Have you seen the duty list? I've got a surprise for you.'

CHAPTER SEVEN

My fury at having to do Madley Out-Patients' turned into rumbling paranoia when I heard that I was also to work as an assistant to Roger Ashe. I had heard Harriet say that he had had three junior doctors working with him in eighteen months: two of them had left the hospital rather than put up with him and one, Dr Singh, had said after a few months of Roger that he would write to the Regional Hospital Board if he didn't get transferred.

It was easy to understand Ashe's unpopularity. Along with an intellectual arrogance that rankled with the other consultants, none of them of any great cerebral ability, Ashe was a snob in the grand manner and made no effort to disguise his colour prejudice. His dislike of Africans and Indians amounted to a phobia; he once told me that every time he thought of the frequency with which another coloured child was born he shook with rage.

I liked the Indian doctors who came to fill the unpopular posts in the hospital, and I found that their gentle ways and efforts to assimilate Western culture were rather touching. I used to dread it when Ashe came into the dining-room and kept up an audible commentary about the smell of oil, the outlandish way the coloured doctors held their knives and forks, and, most serious of all, the liberties they took with something that Ashe held sacred, the English language. He used to collect their verbal *faux pas* and the odd way that they phrased things in the case notes of patients. I can see him now, a tall cadaverous figure with stringy brown hair and pallid skin, crouched in the office of his ward, Watson Ward, and stabbing a long finger at some new horror in the notes.

'Look at this! "Blood transplantations" for "blood transfusions"! And what do you make of this? "A wiry old woman of forty" – I suppose forty is ancient in *their* country. Of course they *can't* pronounce their w's . . .'

Because I had been to the Far East and Ashe had never been farther than France, he used to pepper me with questions about the climate, the noise and the smells. It was beyond him how Asians could settle down in mild England – how could they take to the unflavoured food and the drab dress of the people? He wanted to know the exact difference between Asians and Eurasians, and one of his great sorrows was the fact that the dark gene was dominant, so that every time a fair-skinned blonde married an Indian or an African the result in the progeny was dark eyes and skin. He carried his obsession into his work and I once saw him grab some unfortunate patient and rush her to the windows to see her hands, in case she might have coloured blood. 'It shows in the palms,' he said.

After a chilly period when Roger's off-hand and sometimes cruel attitude to his patients irritated me beyond endurance, I soon found that there were compensations in his uncaring attitude. With Rosie I had been prevented from being involved with the patients because she wanted to make all the decisions herself. I found that because Ashe really didn't give a damn about what happened to the patients as long as there was no trouble and they didn't bother him, I was able to follow up patients from the time they were admitted to the hospital until their discharge.

One morning a girl was sent into Watson Ward after turning up at a police station in the small hours and causing such a disturbance that a doctor was called. The doctor recommended the girl's admission to Bushy Park, and I was called to see her that afternoon because the Sister in charge of the ward, a pretty blonde called Milligan, said that Dr Ashe hadn't been able to get anything out of the patient, who had been given a sedative injection only a few hours prior to admission.

'Anyway, he didn't like the look of her. You know how he is . . . he said there couldn't really be anything wrong with a girl that uses eye shadow.'

Milligan, with her tousled mop of golden curls and huge blue eyes, looked like a doll who might say 'Mama' any moment. Although she appeared as if she had just arisen from a bed of sin, she was very intelligent and had a strong sense of humour. Like me, Ashe's caustic tongue and outspokenness fascinated her.

'I'll see her then, Sister,' I said, and we both went to a small side-room where a girl lay on a narrow bed. She was not wearing make-up – somebody must have washed it off – and, with her long flaxen hair, pale young skin and limpid navy-coloured eyes, she looked angelic.

She was extremely intelligent and I was able to get her to talk about herself without any bother. Her voice had an Irish lilt. Sitting at the side of her bed, I listened to her story with pity and understanding.

She was twenty, she said, and had come originally from a small town outside Cork. The boy she was to have married had deceived her and she had found herself pregnant and penniless. She had been sent to a convent in Dublin by her horrified parents, and there she had had her child in harsh and unsympathetic surroundings. The child was adopted and she had stayed on working in the convent laundry for no money. One night she had gone out to a dance and the nuns had thrown her out. She had come over to England and met a man whom she hoped to marry, but she had found out yesterday that he *was* married, and so she had drunk some gin and become very aggressive. She was sorry, and she regretted causing us all such bother.

Wasn't that just like the nuns, on the scent for sin and yet themselves committing the sin of cruelty? Terry Haynes, the girl sitting quietly beside me, was, I thought, an example of someone who needed compassion and understanding, not censure.

I rushed out and rang the Psychiatric Social Worker, or PSO, who did invaluable work in assessing the social backgrounds of patients and exploring the aids that the National Health Service offered. Mrs Passmore was a stout unpretentious little woman who, after raising three strapping sons, had decided to return to work. She listened to my account of Terry, which sounded even more heartbreaking when I went over it, and promised she would find out what facts she could.

I began to do some work in the ward and Mrs Passmore rang me back in an hour and a half.

'I've found out about Terry Haynes, Doctor,' she said. 'Apparently she's not twenty; she's twenty-seven. She has three children "in care" and she's never been near Ireland.'

There was a pause while I digested this astounding information, then Mrs Passmore coughed and added, 'She's very well known to the police because she's one of Madley's best-known prostitutes.'

'Are you sure?'

'Quite.'

Oh, well, I thought: some you win and some you lose. So much for my gullibility and *naïveté*.

When I tackled Terry about misleading me, she didn't try to wrap anything up. 'Couldn't help it, Doctor . . . I used to love acting.'

Terry was so engagingly frank that I couldn't sustain anger about the deception, and anyway she seemed quite prepared to discuss her occupation, so Milligan and I listened as she told us about herself. She had had a Dickensian childhood, during which her father beat her so hard that she had had several fractures, and after she had reached thirteen he assaulted her sexually and she ran away from home as soon as she could.

'Anyway, Mum died of cancer when she was only thirty-eight,' she added.

She had drifted into prostitution with predictable swiftness and now she was unable to picture a different sort of life. She had a small flat and she went to see her children as often as she could. I noticed the shabby clothes and the battered old suitcase, and I thought that she couldn't be a very successful prostitute, or else she was soft-hearted and didn't overcharge her clients.

What interested me was her almost boastful attitude to her job, and during the next few days I used to go and talk to her as much as I could. I often puzzled over what had become of the prostitutes: we never saw them any more and I wondered if the new sexual permissiveness had interfered with their activity. Terry was unique because she didn't try any more false explanations about herself but admitted that prostitution was the easiest way of making a living; and anyway, she said, I must realize that she *enjoyed* her job. I never quite believed this, possibly because she emphasized it too much or just because she was so highly intelligent. I came across her reading a geometry book one day, and when I commented upon it she laughed lazily and said, 'Am I the first tart you've come across who reads Euclid? I write poems, too, you know!'

She was vague about the events that had led up to her coming into hospital, and I was certain that she had taken drugs on the night of her admission. There was no suggestion of her having had anything to drink and even Mrs Passmore's researches had revealed nothing about alcohol.

'But in that area of Madley, the part where Terry lives, it's easy to get drugs because it's near the docks,' Mrs Passmore told me.

There wasn't much use in talking to Roger Ashe about her. When Terry had been taken in to see him, he only stared at her open nightgown and said frantically to Milligan, 'My God! The view from here! Pin her up, please, Sister.'

One of Roger's peculiarities was that he had a blind spot where sex was concerned and was never prepared to discuss anything below the navel with his patients. It was a joke in the hospital that Roger's one pale child must have been conceived by artificial insemination.

Poor Terry was dealt with smartly by Roger, who told her that she was quite sane and that he couldn't see why she had ever come in to Bushy Park in the first place. When she mentioned that she had taken drugs, he clicked his tongue irritably and said that it was beyond him why a girl of her intelligence should do anything so silly.

I disagreed with Roger about there being nothing wrong with her. Terry's life as a prostitute showed that she had a very low estimation of herself, and the fact that she had to use drugs more and more to keep going made the future grim indeed. I got her to promise that she would stay with us for a while and I decided to have a word about her with the psychologist, Joss Dolan. What Terry needed was prolonged emotional support from someone who was strong enough to deal with her tendency to manipulate, and honest enough not to fob off her questions; and by now I had the highest respect for Dolan's ability. He was adept at establishing a rapport with patients, giving them the chance to develop what was, for many of them, the first healthy relationship they'd ever had.

Dolan was a thin little man with a Punch-like profile and a jockey's build. He was unpopular with many of the doctors because he spoke his mind and made no secret of the fact that to study psychology you needed a higher IQ than you did for medicine. When he came to the hospital he met daunting opposition in his attempts to treat patients. There was a smouldering war between him and the medical staff because the doctors saw the psychologist merely as someone to take intelligence tests, and Dolan simply was not prepared to prostitute his talents in such routine work. He fought back with the tenacity of a ferret, until he wore down the medical staff, who traditionally are unable to keep up an organized and sustained vendetta; and although they still regarded him as a jumped-up busybody who was one of an increasing band of lay people thinking they could do a doctor's job, Dolan was eventually referred enough patients so that he could practise his own brand of psychotherapy. Terry Haynes seemed very suitable material for him, and when I went to his room and told him about her, he dashed to his desk and eagerly opened his appointment book.

'An intelligent prostitute? Sounds like a contradiction in terms, like an honest politician. Anyway, I can see her on Monday. No danger of her being discharged? I don't suppose Ashe cares much, and anyway he won't have a list of patients waiting to come in.'

That was a good thing, anyway. Roger was so uninterested in psychiatry that he kept his clinic very small and didn't encourage GPs to send him patients; if a patient wasn't trouble-some Roger didn't bother discharging him, on the grounds that he might well find himself having to accept someone more troublesome.

When I went back and asked Terry whether she would see a psychologist, she asked me a lot of questions about what a psychologist did, and then she laughed. 'You think I'm a nut case, do you?'

I said I didn't, but I'd like her to do some tests and have a good look at herself with the help of someone like Mr Dolan, who was expert in helping people with their problems.

'Are you trying to pass the buck – I mean, haven't *you* time to sort me out?'

I was used to the necessity of having to explain what a psychologist did, as most people get very confused between a psychiatrist, a psychologist and a psychoanalyst. I told Terry that I wasn't trying to pass her on to someone else in the sense of trying to dump her, but that Mr Dolan had more time than I had and that she would benefit from his help. I didn't add that Dolan was a Doctor, having got his PhD last year, as that often confused people even more.

'And bring your poems. He'll be interested in those,' I added.

I had a phone call from Dolan after he had seen Terry.

'A very interesting girl,' he said. 'I got her to do some per-sonality tests and you know they do show that she's more disturbed than she appears.'

'She says herself that she's a good actress,' I said.

'Well, there's a strong intra-punitive drive in her . . . wants to punish herself for her guilt in hating her father. Of course, being a prostitute is the ultimate in self-degradation . . .'

I had guessed that she was a bit too anxious to tell me that she was happy in her work.

'You know she tried suicide last year?'

Terry hadn't told me that, but I wasn't surprised. So Joss thought she was quite a sick girl?

'I'd like to see her as often as I can for a while,' he said. 'Yes, I do think she's ill, and I think she might try suicide again. She tells me she can buy drugs quite easily. Mind you, today was spent in establishing some sort of rapport with her, which was hard enough as she is quite resistive in a psychic way. Since most of her dealings with men are a sexual trans-action, after which she is able to despise them, she arrived here in a purple trouser suit and did everything she could to seduce me.'

I said that I thought Joss was well able to defend himself, and had she mentioned her poems? He said she had promised to bring them in next time.

'By the way,' he went on, 'what's wrong with Dr Bentley? I passed her on the corridor just now and she was rushing along with some puffing nurse in tow. She told me that she was taking the nurse for an X-ray as she thought she had disc trouble, and then she began to chat about some patient she referred to me. I thought she seemed rather odd . . .'

Trust Joss. Although he didn't move from his little room a great deal, there wasn't much that escaped him; he was like a Geiger-counter for other people's emotional problems. I knew there was no point in trying to kid him, either. I said that for some time Harriet had seemed a bit over-excited to me but that I didn't really know her.

'Well, we'll see,' Joss said. 'Anybody else said anything?'

I said 'No' but I didn't know whether they had observed that the girl wasn't well. Joss said that even if they had, he'd bet that nothing would be said, on the principle that if you ignored something it might go away. In my years of experience of eccentric colleagues I knew that other doctors treat an unstable or drunken practitioner with the greatest tolerance and will cover duty, see patients and act as never-ending stooges rather than do anything that might look as if they were 'shopping' a colleague. The attitude is merciful, but whether it can be said to help a mentally sick person in the long term is a debatable question.

A week after Joss had mentioned Harriet there was a pro-longed ring of my bell one night, and there she stood, wrapped in her black cape and clutching a basket.

'I brought you some peaches,' she said, thrusting the basket at me, and when she came in I took a good look at her while she was taking off her cape. The glitter had gone out of her eyes and there were no circles under them.

'Hey, you do like the peaches? I got some money for doing a cremation and I thought they looked so nice.'

'Indeed they do, Harriet.' I put the soft and very expensive fruit in a bowl, after Harriet had taken one and bit into it so strongly that the juice squirted all over her face.

'Jesus!' She clapped her hand to her mouth and stared at me, bog-eyed. I thought she wanted to clean the fruit juice off and handed her a small towel.

'No, not that. Listen, Joyce, I just remembered something terrible!'

Had she forgotten to take her Pill? Or had she left something burning?

'Oh, Christ! Well, I signed the cremation form yesterday and I put "Yes" in the space where it says "Have you seen the body?"'

I nodded; it was compulsory to view the body if you signed a cremation form. Choking with laughter, Harriet said that she'd meant to go and see the corpse in the mortuary but she had forgotten all about it, and now there was no use bothering because the body would have been taken by the relatives for burial.

'I really meant to go and see the bloody thing but I had to go down to the bank and that put it out of me mind. The thing was, I got a snorter of a letter about me overdraft from the Manager, so I thought, Come on, Harriet, you'll have to do your stuff. So . . . I got into me new turquoise coat – you know the one, it matches me eyes – mind you, it hasn't been paid for yet, but to hell with that! Anyway, I rushed down to the bank and Mr Cowley, the Manager, was just back from lunch, so in I went . . .'

She stood preening in front of my mirror, tossing her hair and looking about twenty.

'. . . and there was this fabulous man. *And* he's a bachelor, *and* he's not queer. I could see he fancied me while I went on about me expenses and how we were all overworked at the hospital. Yes, he said, he understood and certainly I could have me overdraft extended. I stood up and said I had to go because I had to do an operation at three o'clock, and you could see he was impressed.'

Harriet had a habit, when in tight corners, of glancing at her watch and murmuring that she was 'wanted in the theatre'. It was most effective when dealing with policemen or in shops when she wanted to jump the queue.

'Then he asked me to his flat on Saturday. Lives in the West End of Haxton, too.'

Harriet burst out laughing again, and I couldn't help smiling. Her account of vamping the bank manager was adolescent in its *naïveté* and her technique was very unsubtle, but there was a childish and infectious quality about her pleasure which I found amusing. Nobody could use sex and yet make fun of it as well as Harriet.

The idea of having a bank manager amongst her admirers pleased her very much, and as usual she seemed able to rationalize her understanding with Tom. I knew her well enough now to ask whether he knew about her date on Saturday night. She'd lie to him as expertly as she had done to the bank manager.

'Yeah, I'll wear me beige dress and coat— Christ, that reminds me, the dress is rolled in a ball under the bed. I stuck it there the night that fella from the Anatomy Department stayed. Did I tell you about him, Joyce? You wouldn't believe how long he could keep it up. He even wore *me* out, backways, frontways, every way . . .'

My relief that Harriet had regained some stability was very largely due to self-interest. When I was recently qualified I would have enjoyed her dramatics and extravagances unperturbed by the certainty that she was trouble with a capital 'T', that if she ever did have a breakdown she would involve other people. Now I didn't want any more trouble at a personal level. I'd had enough of the challenges in my life. I had been in love, I had had a child and I knew what it was to dread the rustle of bills through the letter-box. For some time now it had seemed sensible to batten down my mental hatches and look at life from the point of view of security for myself and my son. Hadn't I come north to earn more money? I should be glad that Bushy Park hospital was as normal a place as it was, and that apart from the minor kinks of Ashe and Rosie, there were no doctors there with disturbing character traits.

And so I wished I could get rid of the certainty I had that Harriet's return to normality was no more than tremulous, that her 'improvement' was only a brittle and very temporary state.

CHAPTER EIGHT

All the doctors working at Bushy Park had much the same work load, although at times, when the shortage of staff due to leave or illness became acute, we would grumble at having to do extra duty and keep a keen eye on the rota; this important document was pinned every week to the notice-board in the dining-room, and it set out when we were to be on night duty.

The hospital, like most of its type, was three-quarters geriatric, and every doctor had to cover about eight long-stay wards of old people. Since, by virtue of the age of the patients, there were frequent falls, collapses and other emergencies, it meant that there had to be twenty-four-hour medical cover, and we could find ourselves 'on call' for the whole hospital at least once or even twice a week. When on duty, we had to be casualty officer, house physician and house surgeon rolled into one. Very often the patients were so demented that they couldn't help by giving any history, and we had to deal with some blue and panting old lady at two o'clock in the morning, in some back ward, by observing the signs alone. If I say it was like doing veterinary work, I only mean that the poor patients were often as helpless and as speechless as animals.

As well as a quota of back or 'chronic' wards, each doctor attended one out-patients' clinic a week. There were about six of these clinics within the 'catchment area' or radius that the hospital served. The out-patients' clinics were increasing in numbers all the time and served a very useful purpose. By seeing new patients regularly there, we kept the admission rate down, and although Bushy Park took in about eight patients a week, most of those were geriatrics or patients who came under the heading of 'short stay'. If people really had to come in, they often could be accommodated at the flourishing Day Hospital, where they arrived in the morning and went home in the evening.

The basis of any hospital day is the still traditional Doctors' Round. Every morning we started up the long corridor at about half-past nine to see what was going on in our wards. In some, where there were chronic patients, there would be very little doing, but the hard-working nursing staff looked forward to the doctors' round and part of our work consisted in having a cup of tea with Sister and hearing about what went on at the Sisters' meeting, or the pain she had in her back, or something a relative of a patient had said which was upsetting. In listening to the Sister or Charge Nurse of a ward with interest and compassion, we undoubtedly benefited the patients, because psychiatric nursing is a hard, trying and sometimes dangerous slog. Mental nurses are shut up with the patients for hours on end, and their job often shows no dramatic end results; besides which, the ward maid often brings home more money than the hard-pressed nursing staff.

In the old days the young nurses had seemed rather meek creatures, who shook under Sister's glance and were often to be found crying in the sluice room, but I noticed more and more that the youngsters coming from the Nursing School were asking questions and wanting to be involved in more than potting and feeding their charges. They thought about the issues which were formerly regarded as the doctor's province.

Roger Ashe was never done bewailing what he called the 'rise in impertinence' amongst the nursing staff. 'They're not *there* to ask questions,' he said. 'And nurses shouldn't be too intelligent: it makes them bored and disgruntled.'

I didn't agree with him. Certainly a nurse with a Jeeves-like acceptance of her role as a more or less silent recipient of the doctor's orders could make life easier for him, but I felt that since nurses had to face all the dirty jobs, such as cleaning bed-sores, they had every right to ask questions and an equal right to have their opinions listened to.

The nurses at Bushy Park were a kind, hard-working lot, and although the hospital was still rocking from the implementation of the 'Integration Plan' there were now male nurses working on female wards. Women had traditionally worked on male wards for years, but to go into a ward of women and find some strapping young male nurse in charge took some getting used to. Ashe and Rosie had fought a strenuous battle to keep male nurses out of their wards but in the end they had had to give in, causing Ashe to say icily to the unfortunate Deputy Sister on Jasper Ward, 'If I call Sister "Sister", what do I call you – "Brother"?'

One of the things you had to get used to, working in a hospital like Bushy Park, was seeing people die, and it was very often the young nurse who was present at the moment of death. Before the advent of antibiotics, the old patients died quickly after flu and pneumonia, but now there was a huge range of drugs that could be given by mouth or injection, and such patients could rally from what would formerly have been a killing illness. Sometimes you felt in your heart that life was a qualitative thing, and it would be kinder to allow a geriatric patient to slip out of an existence that was lived at a purely vegetable level. Many of our old folk had no relatives, and in spite of all that the overworked nursing staff tried to do, life in the back wards was often a day-to-day monotony of bed pans, rather tasteless meals and the company of other old folk suffering from a variety of physical and mental ills. To see a child was a rarity, and to eat a really fresh bit of fruit depended on whether visitors came. Too often they didn't.

'They put down a dog when he's in pain and going to die, don't they? Well, why has Jane got to suffer so?'

The young nurse who said this to me would have been slapped down by Rosie or Roger, but I thought her question was fair enough and one that I had often thought about myself.

Jane Hart was a skinny patient of sixty-four who suffered from a cancerous ulcer of her face. The malignant sore had eaten away the flesh, and I used to dread coming on the ward when the nurses were dressing the ulcer because I used to have to force myself not to slink by with my eyes averted.

When I started medicine I had been far more able to suffer the sight of decaying flesh. Granted I used to feel pretty terrified inside, but that was more to do with a chronic sense of inadequacy about my ability to be of assistance; I certainly hadn't had to ask the nurses to give me a mask soaked in disinfectant so that I could approach a patient without feeling my guts heave. The sight of Jane's face, with the bone exposed and one eye bulging obscenely on its stalk, was so bad that I wondered how the nurses could bear the awful task of cleaning the wound and dressing it every day. Jane reeked of putrefying flesh, and no matter how often the floors were cleaned with strong disinfectant and the air purified with chlorophyll sprays, the stink lingered. It was better when the bandages were on because they covered the face, making the patient look mummified. One of the most harrowing features was that, as Jane was so confused mentally, we never knew when she was in real pain. I finally told the nurses to give her pain-killing drugs every time she cried, which was pretty often.

The dreadful ulcer had been present for three years now and we all longed for Jane to die, but death was slow in coming – hence the young nurse's heartfelt question.

'I mean, she's on such big doses of morphine that she's going to die of morphine poisoning, isn't she?' the young nurse went on.

'Yes. I'll order such drugs as Jane needs to alleviate pain,' I said, 'but if you mean would I order a lethal dose, then I wouldn't. And even if I did, it would be up to you *not* to give it.'

'But Jane is *rotting* away.' The nurse was a pale, anxious-looking girl who was unpopular with the nursing administration because she was 'difficult', asking searching questions at meetings and writing controversial articles for the hospital magazine. She had twice been turned down for a Sister's post, on the grounds that she wasn't mature. If her queries were an example of immaturity then I had every sympathy with her, because I remembered so well my own anguish at watching suffering and my inability to accept what others seemed to be able to take without soul-searching. In my middle age I had learned how to hide my feelings more, although sometimes I could feel my face muscles harden with the effort to appear calm and professional.

I told the nurse that her question was one which often puzzled doctors and that the answer was impossible to write down with clarity. Although we were not allowed to take life by withholding necessary drugs or giving killing doses, there were situations when it was the right and merciful thing to allow a person to die with some dignity. For instance, I said, if I were called to see a very old patient who was obviously in extremis from some very definite condition, I wouldn't start putting up drips and giving injections into the heart.

'But Jane is dying. Why do you allow her to suffer?'

Jane *was* dying, I explained, but she might last another few months or even a year, and it would be very wrong of me to decide to accelerate her passing. After all – I produced the old argument – in that interval a cure for even a malignancy such as Jane's might be discovered.

The nurse shook her head and I didn't think she was convinced by my answer. I couldn't blame her: a doctor's attitude to death is something that he often doesn't want to discuss, very often probably because he finds it too hard to formulate his views.

'There are things worse than death,' the nurse said, and privately I agreed with her. I wasn't surprised at her next question: Would I tell a patient who had cancer the truth?

That depended, I said. There were very few people who could take the news of their imminent mortality, and usually you found that the more intelligent they were, the more a patient wouldn't ask you the question, because he or she dreaded the answer. On the other hand, there were people who demanded the truth for a special reason, such as the schoolmistress I remembered who had a cancer of her ovary, and who asked to be told how long she had left because she had urgent commitments.

'I believe that if someone really asks you to tell them the truth about their condition, then you ought to respect their wishes and tell them,' I said. 'Sometimes you find that even with the most stable individual, there's a merciful inability to accept the fact that death is near.'

'But I thought most doctors believed that only the nearest relatives should be told?'

I shrugged and said that doctors were nearly all individualists, and good luck to them, but for myself I felt that once you start lying to patients, they have to put up with the indignity of dishonesty as well as their disease, and they end by not trusting anybody.

I wasn't winning her over but at that moment the telephone interrupted me anyway. It was Joss Dolan wanting to talk about Terry Haynes. I said I would go up and see him.

I found him ushering out a boy whom he was seeing for a bad stammer, and as he talked about the patient he rummaged in the drawer of his desk for some papers.

'Terry's poems.' He passed me the sheaf of papers 'They're very good.'

I looked through the poetry. The writing was small and upright and the poetry bleak and depressing. A few pages were headed 'In The Cemetery', and most of the themes were about the harshness of reality which made a drug-heightened world, or even death, more attractive.

'They're all very grim,' I said, but even I, with my scanty knowledge of poetry, could see that the words were expertly chosen and the metre was perfect.

'They're first class, Joyce. We went over some pretty awful material today, a really rough passage. Once Terry ran out of the room, but she came back again. The reason I want to see you is that having stirred up this pool, it's brought a lot of aggression to the surface, and so I think the nursing staff may have to put up with bad behaviour from Terry. Can they take it? And I hope Ashe doesn't order ECT for her . . .'

I said I hoped not. One of the reasons the doctors didn't like Dolan was that he made no secret of the fact that he hated Electro-Convulsive Therapy. Patients he saw would come out with things like 'Mr Dolan said he couldn't see me while I'm having ECT,' or 'I told Mr Dolan that I refused ECT and he said "Good".' Such remarks were guaranteed to infuriate the doctors, who considered Dolan's behaviour unethical and typical of psychologists who weren't bound by a Hippocratic Oath.

'I'll see her again in three days' time,' Dolan said, as he wrote in a notebook. 'You all right?' He had just noticed I was abstracted, half thinking about the young nurse and Jane Hart.

'Oh, I'm thinking about a patient on the back ward,' I said.

'Really?'

Suddenly I was furious with Dolan. Psychologists didn't get the money we doctors did, but they finished their work at half-past four, they didn't work on Saturdays and they hand-picked their patients, rarely bothering about the old, the stupid and the ugly. What they called 'good material' was young, intelligent and attractive patients like Terry. They weren't even around when the patient got really troublesome: the unfortunate nursing staff had to cope then.

'Yes,' I said, rubbing it in. 'She has a cancer that stinks and when you look at it, it's like a bit of meat that's gone bad.'

I saw that he was watching me almost indulgently and I went on, because I wanted to cast Jane from my mind, and tomorrow it was Madley clinic day and I wasn't looking forward to that. I hated Dolan for being able to avoid what I considered the dirty jobs, and I was about to add that instead of holding themselves so aloof from doctors, psychologists ought to do a medical degree and perhaps then they wouldn't be so superior. A few years of the rough and tumble of the back wards, clinics and casualty duty, would soon cut them down to size. After all, if psychiatrists had to study psychology, it was only fair that psychologists should have a knowledge of medicine.

'I hear you go to the Madley clinic now,' he said. 'Is it pretty awful?'

'Yes, it is.'

'Mmmmm . . .' Dolan got up, and a scruffy-looking patient brought in some tea. 'I should think you'll be able to manage the clinic the way you want to soon. It's better than having no clinic. And there's a good attendance as regards patients . . .'

I noticed that there was a big bald patch on Dolan's head and his shirt collar was frayed. My fury disappeared. Joss worked every minute of his time in the hospital and he sometimes was honest enough to say that he thought he could do nothing for a patient, something very few doctors would admit.

'Sorry, Joss,' I said. 'I just feel annoyed.'

There was no need to go on. That was one of the nice things about Joss; he accepted the fact that you got angry and neither pretended you were your usual self nor pried into the reasons. He was also one of the few people who really listened to what you said, and I knew that my surface brittleness and smokescreen of jokes didn't fool him for one moment.

'You really do trail your coat,' he said to me once. 'It's easier to laugh about yourself first before other people have a chance to try it.'

In Watson Ward I found Sister Milligan giggling over the notes Roger had made about some of the patients he had seen that morning.

'This patient is as mad as a hatter and very dim, apart from her insanity.'

'Her husband wants this patient for the weekend, which proves he must be as mad as she is, and I think it is a case of folly *à deux*.'

'There is nothing mentally wrong with this patient. She is a bad lot and should never have been sent to a mental hospital.'

It had been a terrible morning, Milligan went on. One patient, a stout woman who got comfort from the bottle, was so annoyed when Ashe asked her whether she had ever got treatment for her drunkenness that she had darted under the table and bitten him on his elegant calf. I must say I felt a certain sympathy for the goaded woman, because for him an illegitimate child was always a 'bastard', and alcoholism 'drunkenness'. Once we had to take a crippled girl in to the ward and Ashe referred to her in his notes as ' The Incubus'.

The nursing staff liked Ashe's regular routine and his habit of doing his work quickly and without fuss. He didn't hide his lack of interest in the patients and his boredom with the work and he often maintained that the poor nurses had a ghastly job, they were overworked and underpaid. Whenever there was a hint of trouble, therefore, Ashe backed his nursing staff soundly, and I had heard him deal with 'difficult' relatives in a way that was cruelly effective.

If the patient was suffering from the psychosis of schizophrenia, a disease in which the thinking processes become disturbed, he would interview the relatives, and if they got too cheeky or asked too many questions, or complained about the way their mother, daughter or wife was treated, he would lean forward and say, 'Do you realize that schizophrenia is a *hereditary* disease? That it is *genetically* transmitted? Now *I'm* not responsible for your genes, *you* are.'

If they ventured to pursue the conversation and inquire about whether there was a cure, Ashe would say, 'If I knew the cure, I would use it. Nobody knows the real *cause* of schizophrenia so therefore we can't talk in terms of a cure.'

When a patient was really troublesome and the relatives complained about the hospital and the ward, Ashe played his trump card. It was all made more effective by his peculiar death-head face and burning brown eyes.

'If you don't like the way your relative is being treated, then you have the remedy: you can take her home.'

I never got used to Ashe's callousness. I hoped that some of it was unconscious, but there were too many times when patients left his office in tears, and he never bothered to walk up the ward to see what was going on.

I found Terry sitting on the edge of the bed talking to Sally Bruce. Sally was a pale spiky girl who had been in the ward for over a year and showed no signs of wanting to go out. Her childhood had been as bad as Terry's, but she lacked the other girl's intelligence and gained revenge on life by swallowing pins, bolts and needles. Her abdomen was a mass of scars from her operations and the slightest stress made her tremble violently and go off food for days at a time. She was rather a pet of the nursing staff, mainly owing to her habit of climbing on their laps and sucking her thumb whenever she got the chance. Sometimes when I called at the Secretary's office at the front of the hospital, I would find Sally curled on a chair or in somebody's lap, like a small alley-cat.

'You always find someone worse than yourself,' Terry said, as Sally stood on one leg looking at me and then scurried out.

I told her that Mr Dolan thought she wrote good poetry and Terry looked pleased. He was the first man who ever really *talked* to her, she said, and she found that she was telling him all sorts of things she had never told anybody before.

'You feel he's helping you?' I asked.

'Yes, I do. He's done a lot of tests on me and he says I'm very intelligent. I always thought I was a dumbo.'

'Most prostitutes *are* pretty dim.'

She nodded and I thought that that would be the way to attempt rehabilitation, to appeal to her grey matter.

'I guess so. Did I tell you I've always wanted to be a nurse?'

I let that one go, because lots of patients became enamoured of the nurses' uniform and said that they wanted to do nursing.

As I was going out, Sally sidled up to me and pressed a note into my hand. I was going to read it when I got upstairs, but was spotted by Rosie tramping around her sitting-room, which opened on the same corridor as the dining-room. 'I've lost my bloody cheque-book,' she growled.

Rosie's attitude to money was famous: she had inherited a handsome sum from her father who, knowing his Rosie, had left it in trust, and there was her monthly salary, which she never spent. Apart from sweets and cigarettes, her needs were simple. She chucked her bank statements away without reading them, and Roger Ashe claimed to have found share certificates in her waste-paper basket. Roger was wealthy, too, but his money was invested prudently and he watched it accumulate with miserly satisfaction. He was very mean, and he told me once that rather than throw out the free samples of drugs, he sold them to friends. Rosie, on the other hand, was so generous that she gave all her nursing staff crates of drink at Christmas and magnificent presents for all the doctors who worked with her.

'I'm going to the accountant,' she rumbled, 'and he'll *eat* me – oh, here it is!' She rooted down the side of a chair and pulled out a crumpled cheque-book. Although she was going to leave in three months, she had done nothing about her affairs and, as usual, the accountant, who had heard of her leaving from the other doctors who went to him, had had to contact her himself.

'Asking me all sorts of questions about my pension and that,' Rosie grumbled. I knew that she had no idea of what her pension would be.

She was already packing up things. She stood helplessly in the middle of the cases and boxes in this room where she had lived for so long and I thought I could see her eyes glistening. I suddenly realized how I would miss her, and more important, how her patients would miss her. To take her mind off things I handed her the note Sally had scrawled, and was relieved to hear her trumpeting laugh.

'Dear Doc,' she read out. 'Last time I was out I took my small brother into a public lav. I held him over the lav basin and flushed the chain to see what would happen. Nothing did and I brot him home. I think all sattyrisists stink but you are not bad.'

CHAPTER NINE

Doing a clinic for another doctor who is ill can be maddening. The Other Doctor, as the staff call your predecessor, always has different ways from yours. He starts seeing the patients at two o'clock when you like to start at one-thirty, and if you use a particular appointment system then you may be sure he will favour another. He may have a cavalier habit of telling patients to come up *without* an appointment, so that you flounder miserably without case notes to guide you while the patient rapidly loses confidence.

An out-patients' clinic consists of ten to twenty patients, sometimes more, who come at regular intervals to be seen by the consultant psychiatrist. On their first visit their GP sends a letter about them and expects to get a letter back from the psychiatrist. When you try to do letters to GPs at the Other Doctor's clinic, you find that either he likes to do them at the end of the session instead of directly after seeing the case, or that he doesn't dictate them at all but speaks into a tape recorder and has them typed later.

I had covered enough out-patients' clinics for colleagues to know all the pitfalls involved, but up to the time I went to Madley I had never done any clinics for a long period. It was knowing that I'd be doing Madley for a few months anyway (Ellison's doctor was keeping him off duty for six months) that enabled me to arrange everything, including the appointments, the tea, and the letters, to my liking. Best of all, I knew that I wasn't just seeing the patients on one occasion but was going to be able to 'follow them up' for a considerable period.

On my second visit to Madley I arrived wet from a torrential shower that made my hair feel like the coat of a damp spaniel. There was some peculiarity about the rain in Madley; it was always *greasy*.

Mrs Sweetman was on the phone and made a wry face when she saw me.

'She's just arrived. Yes, I'll tell her. Yes.' She hung up. 'That was Mrs Condron, Doctor. She'll be a bit late because the baby has a cold.'

I said that was all right and told Mrs Sweetman to send in the first patient.

'Mr Peter Brooker, Doctor.'

The GP's letter was brief but hopeless. Mr Brooker had an unhappy marriage and had lost his job as a draughtsman with a big firm because of his drinking. He was an intelligent man, wrote Dr Bell, but seemed to be intent on making his life into a terrible mess. 'He is very articulate so will tell you all about himself,' Bell had added as a postscript.

The man seating himself in front of me was a seedy fifty. His face was dusty pink, and when he took off his squashed hat and placed it on the desk I noticed that his plump white hands had a tremor. His stained camelhair coat and scuffed suede shoes made him look like a bookie about to welsh, and his pale blue eyes were watery and shifty.

'Very nice to have a *lady* doctor.'

His teeth, when he broke into what I can only describe as a 'leer', were badly stained.

'Now what seems to be the trouble, Mr Brooker?'

With a deep sigh and a semi-groan, he began to talk about the tragedy of his life. He had been all right while he was in the Army during the war, and when he was demobbed he got a very good job with a well-known firm in Madley. All had gone well until his weakness for women had led him to make the vital mistake of his life: he had married his present wife.

'She caught me on the rebound after I'd been let down by the girl I really loved. I'll tell the truth, Doctor. When I met the wife I'd been drinking heavily for weeks and I wasn't sleeping, even after taking three or four pills a night. I don't know what came over me but Pamela, that's the wife's name, used to be a nurse, and of course at the time that's what I needed – nursing – so we got married. The worst thing I ever did ...'

Half an hour later I was staring at Mr Brooker, having decided that there was really nothing the matter with him, apart from the fact that he seemed unable to cope with life and probably was the sort of inadequate personality who sought in marriage the remedy for his own deficiencies. His wife never bothered to cook, he had told me; their three children weren't properly fed, and although the physical rights of marriage were denied to him because Pamela said she was frightened of getting pregnant again and was afraid to use the Pill, he had followed her and was certain that she was having an affair with a man who lived nearby.

'Not that she's any beauty,' he had added. 'No teeth, and sometimes she doesn't *wash*. But I found out early on, Doctor, that Pamela is a nymphomaniac, she's never satisfied. Oh, there's another thing – she's dog mad. The latest caper is that she's filled the house with three big greyhounds, and she'll cook for the dogs but won't bother to get me a cup of tea.'

Really Mr Brooker's story was sad, but only he had the remedy, to separate and soldier on. I now shifted the subject to his losing his job because of drink.

'I don't deny that I drink to excess,' Mr Brooker cried. 'But when the home life is ghastly what's a man to do? And I can tell you, Doctor, that I'm *liked* in the pub I frequent. The landlord gets me to do his crosswords for him, and I like to demonstrate mathematical problems to people. I don't want to boast but I'm very good at mathematics.'

I said that I believed him. Lack of brains was certainly not Mr Brooker's trouble.

After Mrs Sweetman had come in twice to remind me that there were three other patients waiting, I said to Mr Brooker that I couldn't find anything psychiatric the matter with him and that I would be writing to his GP. Was there any chance of his getting his job back?

'You could help me there, Doctor,' Mr Brooker said eagerly, 'if you ring Dr Dixon – he's the doctor at the works. Here's the telephone number . . .' He scribbled down a number on a piece of paper and passed it to me.

'Right. Now about your next appointment . . .'

I knew I should be firm with Brooker and not give him another appointment. Rosie would have snorted and called him 'a wet'; Roger Ashe would have leant across the desk like a bank manager refusing an overdraft and told him with chilly accuracy, 'There is nothing the matter with your brain, Mr Brooker. As for your matrimonial trouble, well, that is a social problem. You are only one of thousands to be in that predicament and, after all, the choice *was* yours. Again, drinking to excess is something only *you* can conquer. Good afternoon.' It was only patients with lunatic courage who dared to face Roger's arctic rejection a second time!

My motives in giving Brooker another appointment didn't do me credit. What with his despairingly seedy clothes and messy self-pity, I couldn't help feeling sorry for him. I knew he would be a psychiatric albatross, especially when he looked at his appointment for three weeks' time and said, dramatically, at the door, 'I'm completely in your hands, Doctor.' Patients who said that never did very well.

When he'd gone I put a call in to the number he had given me.

'Dr Dixon here.' The voice was brisk and the accent Scots.

I told him who I was and that I had just seen a Mr Brooker who, I believed, had been given the sack.

'Brooker? Oh, aye! An impossible man. Actually the firm have given him *several* chances, Dr Delaney. Did he tell you that?'

'Well . . .'

'He's a most excellent brain. I mean, he's done some first-class work here, but recently he's not been turning in to work, or else arriving half sloshed. I believe he spends most of his time demonstrating his mathematical ability in the local.'

I asked whether he had been really dismissed or whether there was some chance of his being taken back?

'Well . . .' there was a sigh at the other end – 'Brooker behaves like a bloody fool, but when he's sober he's so good at his job that the firm have leaned over backwards to try and help him. Now you tell me that he's going to attend your clinic regularly?'

'He says so.'

'I tell you what I'll do. I'll see the Managing Director and try to get Brooker another chance by telling the Boss Man that he's receiving psychiatric treatment.'

'Thank you very much.'

I put down the phone. At least I'd tried to do all I could for Brooker, and needn't feel guilty when I thought of the three Brooker kids.

Victoria Condron stumped in next, wearing boots and a coat with a fur collar. She sat down in front of me and apologized for being late. I said that was all right and I had got her message.

'The milkman gave me a lift,' she said. 'He's off this afternoon.'

The milkman, it transpired, was a great friend of hers. There was nothing funny about the friendship, she added. The milkman had a wife who was in hospital with nerves and he understood Mrs Condron's trouble.

'Here, why can't you call me Vicky?' Mrs Condron had a knack of making everything sound like an ultimatum. I was surprised that she had come back after the previous stormy interview. Now I had to find out what was really the matter with her. It was evident that she was tense and edgy and she told me that she woke early in the morning and often cried to herself during the day. Her husband was on shift work, and although he gave her enough money the marriage was unhappy because she was frigid.

'And your physical health is good?' I asked.

'Except for my "turns".'

Damn, I'd forgotten that she suffered from a mild form of epilepsy.

'That's why the child is in a nursery and I can't have any more children,' she said. 'I looked up all about epilepsy in a book but they don't tell you what it's really like. Mind if I smoke?'

I said 'No' and she whipped out a paper parcel and began to unwrap it. It was a white china ashtray. 'A present for you,' she said. I thanked her and listened to how the seizures affected her life.

'I hate being alone,' she said. 'That's why I make a huge pot of tea so as to keep the milkman as long as possible. Then I have to force myself to go out. I'm terrified of shopping since I had one of my turns in Woolworth's and I passed out on the floor, but as I was coming round someone stuck a rolled cloth into my mouth and I heard some woman say that that was what you did to epileptics, so as they won't bite their tongues. And an ambulance brought me home. Even if I do manage to get out, there's that afternoon to put down. We have a small bungalow so there's nothing much to do as regards housework. I listen to the wireless a lot and I turn on telly, even when there's only the test card.'

'Haven't you any friends?'

'On the estate they're mostly out working, or else they've got young kids. And I'm always afraid of passing out. I did that once in a friend's house and her little daughter was so frightened she screamed her head off. You don't know how awful you feel when you've got something like me, it makes you different . . . a freak.'

She pulled out her handkerchief and cried for a bit. Although her tablets helped to cut down her fits, she still had one or two every week, and they were frightening because she always lost consciousness. When she woke up she only had a hazy memory of the events leading up to the attacks.

I had never really liked dealing with epileptic patients; they often have an explosive, unattractive temperament, with irritable dispositions to match their overcharged brains. But as I listened to Vicky the real practical difficulties of the disease dawned on me. With most other illnesses you could share your symptoms with other people, but epilepsy was different. Having a fit was essentially a lonely and personal business. She had had a turn on the bus once, and this was why she had to take taxis to collect her small daughter from school.

'Would you mind if I asked a Mental Welfare Officer to call on you?' I asked.

Vicky said that she wouldn't mind anybody calling, so when she went out I phoned the Mental Health Office and arranged a meeting with the MWO on duty, a Mrs Redmond. She could come up in half an hour. First I had to see the Tasker family again.

Mr Tasker was in command, as usual, directing the disposal of coats and propping up the baby on the examination couch.

Ambrose had been off school for over a week, he began, pointing to his son, who looked as if a strong breath would blow him away. Although he, Mr Tasker, had written a full explanatory letter to the school, a very nasty man from the Education Department had turned up at the house and been rude. As he noticed that the caller hadn't got good grammar and he thought he detected a smell of beer on his breath Mr Tasker had put his coat on and gone himself to the Education Department to complain.

'I was shown in to the Head of the Department, an intelligent man with perfect manners. It proves what I always say, Doctor: you only get real rudeness from men of little ability. I was given an apology and an assurance that it wouldn't happen again.'

I made suitable congratulatory noises, and then Mr Tasker stabbed a finger at his wife. 'You've not been well at all, have you, Annie?'

His wife was fiery red and asked if he could open some window. While he struggled with the stiff catch, she told me about the horrible attack she had had four days ago.

'I thought me end had come, didn't I, Amby?'

The boy stopped twiddling his skinny thumbs and nodded mutely. God help him, I thought, sandwiched between Father's endless guerrilla warfare with bureaucrats and Mother's brushes with death.

'Yes. I came over all cold and I could hear my heart pounding, pounding. Harold was out at work, so when the room began to go round and round, I got Amby to help me up to bed and see to the baby.'

I tried unsuccessfully to picture the boy supporting his vast mother.

'Anyway, when Harold came in he said I ought to see the doctor, so I made my way down to the surgery only to find that Dr Jones had had to go to a funeral and there was a locum there, an old man, and he was deaf as a plant because when I told him about my attack he said, "Good, good, that's what we like to hear!" He must have thought that I was feeling well! He gave me some tablets to take and ... you better tell the rest, Harold.'

The baby woke up and began to wail. Mrs Tasker snatched it up and retrieved its dummy, which appeared to be suffocating it.

'I'm in the habit of examining tablets,' Mr Tasker said. 'Curiosity, as you might say. Well, while I was waiting for Mrs Tasker I was reading a medical magazine and there was an advertisement for the same tablets as my wife had, which said, "The ideal pill for the troublesome patient." Well, I mean! ... Annie could have asked the doctor to *call*, but she was only trying to make things easy ...'

And so it went on, this family forum for discontent. I decided to make it a long interval before their next appointment and expected ructions, but surprisingly Mr Tasker didn't object. The reason for this became clear as they were about to go.

'I know you're very busy, Doctor,' he said. 'The waiting-room's *full* of other unfortunates, but, I wonder, would you be kind enough to see our nephew, Cedric. His nerves are in a shocking state.'

'Would he be willing to come?'

'Oh, yes, he's perfectly willing. Why, when we were talking about how nice you were to us, Cedric said that's just what he needed, a sympathetic doctor.'

I said to tell Cedric that I couldn't see him without his being referred from his own doctor, and Mr Tasker admitted that Cedric's doctor would be only too anxious to get rid of him. Cedric had come home in tears last time because of the rudeness he had suffered at Dr Slattery's surgery.

Everyone knew that Dr Slattery, a huge Kerry man with such a violent temper that one infuriated patient had set his Alsatian dog at him, hated neurotic patients. I could imagine the barracking he must have given Cedric.

'I don't want to call one doctor to another, and I know that Dr Slattery comes from your own country, but Cedric said that the language Dr Slattery used was disgusting.'

I could believe *that*. I'd heard how Slattery had once rushed into his waiting-room to find out why all the patients were going to see his partner.

'Anyone for me?' he had yelled at the trembling gathering. 'Well f— the lot of you!'

We all wondered how Tim Slattery escaped being reported to the General Medical Council.

Mrs Redmond turned out to be a handsome woman with a personality as ample as her body. She listened to my description of Vicky and said that she would call and bring the girl to the Young Wives' Association.

'It seems a bit hard that she has to depend upon the milkman for company. Actually I'm glad you rang, Doctor. Mr Cox – he's the chief of the department – and I were wanting to meet you. How are you getting on? Mrs Sweetman says that the patients are increasing. I think that the GPs have heard there's a new doctor at the clinic, and as you're a woman they'll probably send you all their troublesome females. Now I have a woman I'd like you to see, Doctor. She used to be a patient in Bushy Park and I've been keeping an eye on her since her discharge. She's a strange woman. You won't think I'm daft?'

'Indeed not.' Mrs Redmond was patently sane.

'Well, I think this woman has some sort of psychic power. She's a seventh child of a seventh child and she lives in a remote little village where everybody seems to be frightened of her. Her husband is a big boor who spends most of his time drinking. The patient, a Mrs Denning, hates him.'

'Why doesn't she leave him?'

'Well, he earns good money. I don't think she'll leave him as long as he's working, but when he retires ...' Mrs Redmond paused. 'You'll have every reason for thinking that I'm dotty, but I sometimes think that Mrs Denning will poison him. Even now he gets mysterious stomach upsets after he's been particularly trying.'

I began to look forward to seeing Mrs Denning and I told Mrs Redmond to bring her along next week.

When I got back to the hospital I called in the small room where our mail was put, as I had forgotten to collect my letters that morning. Roger Ashe was sitting at the table, lugubriously tearing up a pile of advertisements.

'Oh, hallo, Joyce,' he said. 'I've just had to order a sedative for that little tramp Terry Haynes. D'you know she had the cheek to ask me why I had taken up psychiatry? I nearly said for the same reason you took up prostitution ... Anyway, she's been seeing Mr Dolan – he *always* makes patients cheekier – and of course when Sister rang him he had gone home.'

'Is Terry going home?'

'I'd hoped she would, but she wants to see Dolan again. He should watch out, you know; a girl like that could make allegations. He hasn't had a medical training or he'd make sure he was chaperoned with that type of patient.'

It was a relief that he didn't appear to have put a veto on Terry's visits to Dolan and that she hadn't insisted on taking her discharge, though I was glad when he changed the subject. He had felt like some tea after visiting the ward, he told me, but to his annoyance had found Dr Ishraf in the dining-room vetting the sandwiches, prying them open and slapping them together again. Ishraf was a vast man who had come to us a month ago to take a registrar's post. He was rather stupid, if amiable, and would not be put off by Ashe's sniffs and sarcasm. He constantly chattered to him about the weather and whether Ashe thought his English was coming along.

Trying to ignore a strong smell of Gorgonzola cheese, Ashe was about to sit down at the table and drink his tea when he noticed that Ishraf was now lying back in his chair, with his huge stockinged feet on the table. Ashe had remonstrated with him and insisted, not unreasonably, I thought, that he put on his shoes forthwith, because in England it wasn't done to take your shoes off in public.

'What did he say?' I asked.

'He beamed and asked me what "forthwith" meant!' Roger groaned. 'Oh, Joyce, I give up! Why *can't* they all go back to their own country?'

CHAPTER TEN

The next morning I made my way up to Watson Ward as soon as possible and asked for Sister. As I expected, I found that Milligan was off and her relief was a charge nurse called Brown, whom I disliked intensely for being stupid and a liar. She had a shiny face and pop eyes, and when she wasn't shouting at the patients she sat in her room smoking furiously.

'Yes, Terry Haynes has been terrible.' She shoved the report book at me and tapped an entry which read, 'Haynes refused to go to bed when told and became very aggressive. Used foul language. Had to be given a second sedative.'

We found Terry chatting quietly to a girl who had come in to us the week before, after she had tried to kill her new-born baby. I asked Terry to come into the office at the end of the ward, and when the three of us were seated in the room I questioned her about the episode of the previous night.

'I *did* answer back,' she said. 'I was feeling a bit upset after seeing Dr Ashe. Does he *have* to be so cold? My God, it's like trying to talk to a corpse! Well, there was a good play on TV and I was looking forward to seeing the end when I was told to go to bed – not asked, *told*.'

She glared at Sister, who glared back.

'So I just sat tight, and then Sister called me a selfish street-walker who was taking up a bed needed for someone else.'

'I *never*!' Sister Brown shouted.

I decided privately that she might well have been tactless in dealing with Terry, but I certainly didn't want a shouting-match now, so I told Terry that rules were rules and bad language wasn't the way to make your point.

'Well, I only do it when someone calls me first,' Terry said.

Trying to change the subject, I told her that she should be thinking of a job, and why didn't she see one of the social workers with a view to getting a job?

'Are you trying to get rid of me?' She was so insecure that she was always on the defensive. I said that I wasn't trying to push her out at all, but I didn't want her to get too 'dug in'. Many of the patients took to the safe and undemanding life in the sheltered atmosphere of the hospital, and put off trying the outside world for too long.

'Terry is displaying aggression now,' I said to Dolan when I telephoned him later.

'That's healthy. The nursing staff must learn to cope with it,' Dolan said.

But I knew that only the more intelligent nurses would realize that a show of spirit like Terry's cheek could be a normal and proper resistance to the institutionalization that goes on in every large hospital.

'I hope Terry keeps contact with you,' I said. 'I have an awful feeling that she'll go back to being a prostitute.'

'We've got to take that risk,' Dolan said.

'I've told her to get cracking about a job,' I said. If I analysed my motivation in telling him this, it was because I resented what I thought was his great fault, that of making patients overly dependent upon him. I argued with him about this sometimes, but he brushed it aside by saying that in any relationship between a therapist and a patient you had this obstacle, and the thing to do was to acknowledge it by open discussion with the patient, what Dolan called 'Working through the Positive Transference'. The other doctors got incensed with his complete take-over of a case, but all I felt was an occasional impulse to demonstrate that I, too, was still interested.

'Rather early, don't you think, to be considering a job for her?'

I knew he would say this, so I was ready for it. I told him

that Ashe was already annoyed with Terry, as was Sister Brown, and that if the girl showed any more agitation she might well be given ECT.

'It's incredible ... to use that bloody box as a weapon,' Dolan said. The loss of memory and confusion following the treatment always made the patient unsuitable for psychotherapy, hence Dolan's dislike of it.

In the end my admiration for him always triumphed over my irritation, so I threw him a verbal bouquet. 'Anyway,' I said, 'I think Terry is *much* better.'

The same morning I met Dr Hedley talking to an MWO in the corridor. He made a sign for me to stop and said, 'Could I see you a minute, Dr Delaney?'

I followed him into his office and listened as he took up the ringing telephone.

'The voices are telling her what? OK, Doctor, I'll be around in about half an hour. Yes. OK.'

He scribbled an address on the pad in front of him. An important part of a consultant psychiatrist's work is in going out to see mental patients in their own homes, at the request of the GP or the MWO. These domiciliary consultations or visits, commonly known as 'DVs', may sometimes result in the patient being sent into hospital, either by putting him on a certificate or 'section', if he is unwilling to go in voluntarily and is a danger to himself or others; or, as is more common these days, the patient would come in on an 'Informal' basis and could leave whenever he liked. If hospitalization wasn't considered necessary, the psychiatrist might make an arrangement to see the patient at an out-patients' clinic or might, in the case of a very old patient, put his name down on the ever-increasing list for geriatric beds. It happened sometimes that the unfortunate patient seen on the domiciliary visit died before a bed could be found for him.

'Two things,' Dr Hedley said, after he had taken another phone call. All conversation with Hedley was punctuated by the phone and by nurses wanting to speak to him. He was at the opposite end of the scale to Ashe. While Roger spent as little time as possible in the wards, pruned his clinic to the minimum and refused to do any DVs by being so frosty to the GPs that they never asked him, Hedley was in the hospital from nine in the morning to seven at night, after which he did his domiciliary calls. As a result he never got home before ten. Although he suffered from bad bronchitis and had an invalid wife, poor Hedley's milk of human kindness was doubly rich, and he got all the boring chores that nobody else wanted, such as acting as secretary to innumerable committees, and examining nurses.

I liked Hedley. He wasn't amusing and he looked rather like an ant-eater, but although he worked so hard he was always ready to help if you were in difficulty, and rather than call another doctor he would deal with everything himself.

Dr Ellison would be away for the full six months, he told me, and Dr Sanders had just found that she had got more time in than she thought, which meant that she could retire sooner than she had allowed. That was typical of Rosie. She was so vague about anything that involved writing or phoning that two years ago she discovered she had managed to get herself off the Medical Register through not answering a letter from the General Medical Council, and she had been practising illegally for a few months. Dave Hedley had to sort things out by writing to the GMC on her behalf.

'So what I'd like to know is whether you would be prepared to "act up" and do consultant's work until we make a new appointment?'

I said I would like to very much. I wouldn't make much more money, apart from the fee that you got for DVs, but the work would be more interesting.

'OK. I'll ask the Regional Board. I'm sure they'll agree ... Now, the next thing is, we've got to arrange a present for Rosie Sanders. She is now going in a week or two. Do you know what she would like? I'm sure all the doctors will want to contribute. She's been at Bushy Park for so long ...'

I was less pleased about having to ask Rosie what she wanted as a farewell present. I had an idea that the change of plans wouldn't improve her temper – the prospect of having to run a house, small though it was, and coping with shopping and cooking, depressed her and made her edgy.

There was no use looking for her until the evening, because she was always either at her clinic or stuck down in her wards, so I waited until after supper – it was always best to pick a time when she had eaten – and went up to the doctor's dining-room, where I found Rosie curled in her favourite armchair and positively glowing after what she said was a very good supper. She patted her stomach contentedly.

Cashing in on her mood, I sat down beside her, and watched her play Patience. Her fat square hands moved surely and rapidly, slapping down the cards at which she barely looked. When she came up from the wards she played Patience for hours. I decided it would be tactless to go on about my being asked to 'act up', so I waded right in and asked her what sort of present she would like. She swept up the cards rapidly.

'Now you can tell Hedley that I want nothing,' she said unhesitatingly. '*Nothing*. I know all the silly nonsense that goes on at these presentations, and I always swore that I wouldn't have one. It's just another way of being—'

At that moment Harriet crashed in, carrying her black cape over her arm and looking as if she hadn't slept for weeks. Rosie seized on her entry to get over her embarrassment about the present. She had been much nicer to Harriet in the past few weeks, since the girl had been put on some of her wards. Rosie was always quick to appreciate anyone who cared about the patients. Now she decided that Harriet should have some of the strawberries left over from dinner and she pattered out to the kitchen.

'I'm on duty.' Harriet delved into her bag, looking for her cigarettes. 'I was called to see a man in Singh's ward. He was admitted two days ago and Singh hadn't written a line about him. He's a sod, you know, Singh: clever but lazy. Hey, did I tell you about going out to see the bank manager? Well, he has this huge pad with the moddest of cons in every room, really fabulous. He cooked gorgeous steak and then we had two bottles of wine.'

She laughed loudly, and the sound went on too long. She looked haggard and distraught again, her eyes shadowed and her forehead sweaty. I noticed that her hair had lost its shine and the collar of her blouse was grubby. As she chatted on about the ardour of the bank manager, I wondered at his indiscretion in making a date with a customer like Harriet, and then it occurred to me that the average individual trusted doctors.

When Rosie returned, Harriet took the large bowl of strawberries and cream from her and spooned them quickly into her mouth.

'I was just thinking, folks,' she said, putting down the empty bowl and not bothering to wipe the fruit juice from her mouth, 'what about us having a party? We could give it in this room and I'll bring in me records. I've got a few fabulous tapes. We'll have old Tom as barman and we'll slip Roger a Mickey Finn ...'

'No, you won't, dear, because he won't come,' Rosie said. 'His wife is "agin" parties, and she'd be more agin them if she caught sight of *you*, Dr Bentley!'

Harriet was delighted. 'Hey, do ya think I'm sexy, Rosie? Could ya tell from looking at me?'

Shaking with laughter, Rosie began to slap down the cards.

'You, Harriet, have a sign around your neck saying "Available", that's what you have, a sign around your neck!'

Harriet took out her handbag mirror. 'Oh, God, do ya think I'm developing dewlaps?' She wobbled her chin. 'I often think I'm a nympho, can't seem to get enough sex. Mind you, I might as well use what I've got when I can, mightn't I? I went out to a strip show with a fellow last week, and afterwards he made me do all sorts of things ... he tied me wrists and that ...'

She jumped up to answer the phone, smoking her cigarette in short useless little puffs. I saw Rosie staring at her and I knew that she had noticed Harriet's mood.

'Have to go, folks,' she shouted. 'I'll have a good think about the party. It's about time we got something going in this place ... it's like a morgue. The maids wouldn't mind doing us sanis, would they? And I know a place where you get very cheap booze. See ya ...'

But she'd forgotten her cape and it was when she came running back for it, panting heavily, that I noticed her swollen ankles. She caught me staring at them.

'Oh, yeah, me ankles.' She prodded them with one hand. 'I must be getting congestive cardiac failure, mustn't I? I'm breathless, too. Do me ears and lips look blue?' She laughed, but her eyes were desperate.

'Get a good sleep tonight,' Rosie said.

'Sleep? You just *have* to be joking, kid. I only sleep about *two hours a night*. Can't get off. Hey, must say tatty-bye, there's a patient aborting and I may have to put up a blood drip.'

When she had gone clattering noisily down the stairs, I said to Rosie, 'What do you think? She's very ill, isn't she?'

Rosie smacked down her cards, looked at them and then swept them up again. 'That girl,' she said, 'is on drugs. I've seen it before. She's taking drugs and you, Joyce, must have a jolly good talk to her. You're older than she, and if she goes around looking and talking the way she is, God knows what trouble she'll get into. And think of the damage she's doing to our image.'

I wondered whether Harriet was able to cope with being on duty, and yet I knew she would throw out any suggestion that she wasn't fit to work. I wished that I was as certain as Rosie about the cause of the girl's instability.

'It's your duty,' Rosie said, when I didn't respond. 'I'm going any day now, you know.'

CHAPTER ELEVEN

I soon found out that I would get no practical help about Harriet from the other doctors either. At the end of lunch the next day, after Rosie had gone to her clinic and the others at the table were talking about the rise in the number of abortion requests, she trailed in clutching a bulging handbag. Her eyes looked enormous and her cheeks were very red. If you hadn't known her you might have thought she had been drinking, but there was no smell of drink.

'Hi, folks! Any grub left?'

She sat down beside one of the younger doctors, Toby Mason, and looked around. 'Never mind, I'll just have a cup of coffee. You haven't got foot-and-mouth disease, have you, Toby?'

Before he could say anything she had snatched his used cup and poured coffee into it. Then she lit a cigarette and said loudly to the other doctors, 'Listen, everybody ... I'm going to organize that party. Everybody can give a quid – that'll buy plenty of drink. How about it?' She nudged Toby's well-covered ribs. 'You can give us a bit of the old soft-shoe shuffle, Toby.'

Mason murmured something noncommittal, and she shouted across at Hedley, 'Will you come, Dave? I've got a whole lot of Jeanette MacDonald and Nelson Eddy records ... Just your vintage!'

She burst out laughing and I could see everyone looking at her. Hedley grinned self-consciously, while Singh, with eyes glowing like warm coals, said that he'd love to come.

'And Rog ... live dangerously, old boy, and come and join us ... You can all bring your wives if you like. Mr Whittaker, what about you?'

Mr Whittaker was the orthopaedic surgeon who visited the hospital once a week and came up for his lunch, a period when he spoke of nothing but gardening and his work. He was a thin man with a stammer, and now he glanced round him desperately.

'Party? ... Live so far away ... Must g ... g ... g ... get back to the theatre.' There was a hair-raising pause as he gurgled to get his words out, and then he rose and rushed out.

'That poor guy needs treatment for his stammer,' said Harriet cheerfully, whipping out a notebook and beginning to write rapidly in it. I was opposite her and I tried to make out what her flying hand was writing. Normally she wrote clearly but now the pages were covered with lines of indecipherable squiggles.

Later that afternoon Roger came into the room in the ward where I was writing up notes.

I wasn't working with him since I had been asked to cover Ellison's work, but I had come up to say goodbye to Terry Haynes, who had got herself a job. Having discussed it with Dolan, she was going to try to cope outside the hospital. She thanked me for all I had done, but she and I both knew that Joss was the person who had really helped her. I had only been a sort of liaison officer to make sure that she saw him. I watched her leave the ward and hoped that I wouldn't see her again.

'That girl Harriet is not well,' Roger said, hunching his shoulders and staring out of the window, hands in pockets.

'Oh, she's young,' I said. 'Late nights, too much smoking, finishing her MD thesis.'

'No,' he said. 'More than that.'

'Like what?'

'Well, if she was a patient I'd say she was in mania, or to put it more crudely, she's "high".'

'All right,' I said. 'Any suggestions for what we should do?'

'What can one do?' Roger was horrified. 'It's most unfortunate but it's *her* problem. I would like to know whether she showed anything like this behaviour in her last job. Of course, they mightn't say if they wanted to get rid of her, might they? It's quite dreadful to see the state of her, and you never know what she's going to come out with, do you? All that business about the party ... terribly awkward. I could see Whittaker looking at her – he'll put that right round the Haxton hospitals. She should go off on a long holiday, that's what she should do.'

I could have screamed. Roger didn't dislike Harriet; indeed, after an initial period when her plebeian accent had alarmed him, he had succumbed to her undoubted charm and rather enjoyed the way she rattled on. But he obviously wasn't going to do anything to help her.

'Did you see Mason's face when she said he could do a soft-shoe shuffle?' Roger gave his odd laugh, which was like a seal snorting. 'I wonder how she's managing to do her work. She's so restless it makes concentration difficult.'

The strange thing was that Harriet seemed to be able to cope quite well with her work. A few of the nurses had asked me if Dr Bentley was all right, and probably the more intelligent of the nurses guessed that she was mentally ill, but although she looked as if daemons were chasing her and didn't bother with her appearance, she attended to patients when on duty, wrote clear and legible notes and ordered doses in the right amounts.

I thought at first that I might be able to ask Tom about Harriet, but either he had guessed at last that she was ill and had decided to get out of the situation, or she had let slip about the bank manager or one of her innumerable one-night stands, for she told us one day that Tom had gone back to Ireland for an indefinite period as his mother was ill.

When I came into the residents' sitting-room one afternoon, Singh was there. He put down *Lancet* and gave me one of his flashiest smiles. He was very handsome if you liked slumbrous eyes and teeth.

'I'm afraid that you are missing tea, Dr Delaney. Dr Bentley was being here just before your arrival. She was not saying anything about the party so perhaps she has forgotten about it?'

'Probably.'

So Harriet was in. I went to the notice-board. She wasn't on duty.

'Dr Delaney, don't you think that Dr Bentley is very ill? What do you think is the likely diagnosis? There are features suggesting mania at the moment. She is too emotional to be considered under the heading of schizophrenia. I think she should be on sick leave. Otherwise you will be having the patients discussing her and that will not be good, isn't it?'

'I don't think that Dr Bentley *is* a subject for discussion,' I said stiffly. I knew I had hurt Singh's prickly feelings by the reproachful look he gave me but I was annoyed at his voicing my own thoughts, especially in such bad grammar, and I was fed up with people talking about Harriet without coming up with any practical suggestions about helping her.

I hung around the front of the hospital and at about half-past six Harriet appeared, looking dashing in a red tweed coat with a black fur collar and cuffs.

'Hi, Joyce.'

'Are you on your way somewhere?' I asked.

'Only to rest me feet for a bit. I'm going out later.'

I followed her into the small room where we doctors who lived outside used to leave our coats. She tore off her coat, saying that she was roasting, and flopped into an armchair.

'Christ, look at me feet! I must tell you about the bloke I'm going to meet tonight, Joyce. He's quite old, in his fifties, I'd say, but *very* intelligent. I met him at a university do last week. He's got a grant from the Medical Research Council, you know, to do some work on vaccines. I could sense him staring at me and the next thing, he gets himself introduced to me. Karl Pengle – ever heard of him? Anyway, he told me that he's just recovering from a depression and that didn't surprise me, because even though he's very bright and gives you a sort of *glittering* impression, I would say that he's very, very sensitive. I'm meeting him at the Juniper, you know, the University Club, at eight. How do I look? I bought this coat with the overdraft money!'

'Very nice,' I said mechanically.

Trust Harriet to latch on to some neurotic. A favourite phrase of hers was 'It takes one to know one', and indeed she attracted people with personalities as fragile as her own. Tom was an exception but it looked as if he had baled out for good.

She was humming a little tune as she combed her tangled hair and began to rub on some lipstick. I decided on the direct approach.

'Harriet,' I said, 'you've got very thin, and all this not sleeping – why don't you see someone?'

'Yeah, I *have* got thin.' She opened her coat and pulled out her dress at the waist. 'I don't know ... I may have an overactive thyroid gland, mayn't I?'

Was she deliberately trying to pinpoint a physical cause for her trouble or did she really think that she had an organic illness?

'Are you still taking the Pill?' I asked.

'No. Though that means I have another worry, pregnancy.'

'Anything else? Are you taking any other pills?'

It was out and I knew she understood what I meant by the quick flicker of her eyes.

'I'm not taking anything. I'll be all right when I can sleep again.'

'You look ill.'

I couldn't press the matter of drugs further. I was pretty

sure that whatever the matter was with her, it wasn't drugs.

'I tell you what, I'll fix up to have a full check-up next week. I'll make an appointment with Maxie.'

Maxwell Evans was the consultant physician at the General Hospital in Haxton. I said that was fine and that I would go with her. I thought for a second she was going to tell me to mind my own business but she just gazed in the mirror and said, 'OK. You know, I wouldn't be surprised if Maxie doesn't find lots of things the matter with me, although last year when I was ill . . .'

She didn't finish the sentence and I had to control my curiosity about her previous illness. She had suddenly turned round and was looking at me. Her eyes should have been beautiful because they were large and well-shaped, but the peculiar staring effect and the very deep shadows made her look sick.

'I'm not ill enough to be certified.' She said it very quickly and sharply and before I could say anything she continued, 'Anybody who tries to get me certified will be in trouble, that's for sure.'

When I collected her on Monday at half-past one, she looked perfectly composed and was wearing a new and very short navy dress with a blue and white bow at the neck. She sat beside me with her eyes closed in the car and didn't seem in the least nervous. She must be a very good actress or else she's had a sudden remission in her illness, I thought, as we went into the waiting-room.

Placidly she sucked a sweet and read a magazine while we waited.

'Dr Bentley?' The receptionist looked at me. She must have thought Harriet was my daughter and I didn't blame her, because what with Harriet's long hair, short skirt and a face which today looked positively dewy, she gave the impression of being just out of her teens. Why couldn't she have looked haunted and haggard? Maybe I should have seen Dr Evans first.

She was over half an hour in the consulting room and came out smiling happily. 'Swinging. I'm dying for a fag. And I could do with a cup of coffee and a sani. You know, I don't think Maxie's all that good on hearts. I didn't like the look of my electrocardiograph . . .'

I said that I would like a word with Dr Evans, and before she could say anything I knocked at his door.

He was a tall man with a pale face, good-looking in a glacially patrician way. You could underestimate his skill as a doctor because of his plummy voice and dandified dress, but he was a most able physician, kept himself in touch with modern advances by attending courses at home and abroad, and was always writing for the journals. It was said that he had only come to Haxton because he had offended the Professor at his teaching hospital by questioning a diagnosis.

I said that I was no relation of Dr Bentley but that she seemed to have changed recently and that we were worried about her.

'Ah, yes.' Maxwell Evans looked down at his folded hands. 'A very excitable girl, very emotional. I gave her a very thorough examination and could find nothing. *She* insists that she gets cardiac pain, so just to allay her anxiety I did an electrocardiograph examination and it was perfectly normal. D'you know, she argued the toss with me? Said she could see an inverted T-wave . . .' Maxie laughed rather coldly. Nobody argued with him about hearts, he was a recognized expert.

'What about the ankle swelling?'

'My dear Dr Delaney, the girl doesn't eat. The swelling is due to a vitamin deficiency. I told her that although she's too thin, she is perfectly healthy, but I don't think that I convinced her.'

I hadn't thought that Harriet had anything the matter with her organically, but I was hoping that Maxie would agree with me that the girl needed psychiatric help.

He smiled when I mentioned this. 'A psychiatrist to treat another psychiatrist?' I could see it was no good. I knew that Maxie made little secret of the fact that if psychiatrists weren't mad when they went in to the speciality, it wasn't long until they became so. He shrugged and didn't go on. He didn't need to, I knew what he meant. In the old days Harriet would have been a nursemaid or an intelligent barmaid.

* * *

I wasn't able to see Rosie until the night before she was leaving. I went into her room and found her bawling that she couldn't find her lipstick. I told her to try her bag and sure enough it was there.

'So Maxie is washing his hands of it? Well, we knew there wasn't anything physically the matter with her.'

'Where do we go from here?'

'We don't. Can't do any more now. And from what she said about certification, she knows the score herself. How do I look? I'm going to my presentation from the nurses.'

She looked very well in a gold blouse and black skirt, and I told her so. She pulled down her skirt with her stubby hands and sighed. Thirty years was thirty years, and she had given them all to her patients. A new doctor would come and laugh at her treatments, and some of the nurses who didn't understand her would be delighted that a doctor whom they thought of as a bad-tempered old woman would not be around to run trolleys over their legs and shout at them. Some other nursing staff who were inefficient or stupid would be glad that they were no longer going to have case notes thrown at them, or be made to shiver at one of her shouts.

'Come with me?'

I declined. The nurses wouldn't like me there and it was, after all, Rosie's night.

What would become of all the patients on the Treatments? And the menopausal ladies at the clinics? Who would listen to accounts of the Haxton Flush?

'You know what?' Rosie's voice was wobbly. 'I didn't expect to feel so lonely. I'm going to take something to buck me up.'

I thought she meant a drink, but she pulled out a glass bottle and popped some tablets into her mouth.

'The Pips,' she said. 'They *never* fail.'

CHAPTER TWELVE

After her visit to Maxwell Evans, Harriet did one of her amazing switches to comparative normality and then, telling everyone that she had been advised that she was too thin and generally run-down, disappeared for a few weeks. I heard that she had gone to London on holiday.

Rosie left at last and I was glad that I was kept very busy because I missed her and the slap of her Patience cards. Her clinic was amalgamated with Toby Mason's, and the lamentations of the ladies 'on the change' was long and loud. Indeed, one or two of them were so distraught after Rosie's departure that they broke down and had to be admitted.

I tried DVs with some foreboding, remembering how hard it had been to locate addresses during my stint in general practice, but here an MWO drove me to the patient's home and was able to fill me in on the history and family background. 'It's the Old People who are the most difficult to deal with,' I was warned, and how true this turned out to be.

When I had started psychiatry I had been appalled at the horrors of the geriatric wards in the hospital I was attached to. Toothless, without personal possessions or clothes other than the drab wear that the hospital provided, the old folk inhabited bodies that had outlived their minds, and eked out their remaining days in conditions that used to make me thank God that their mental faculties had left them, for if they had been lucid they would have preferred death. Now, fifteen years later, I saw old people in the community in conditions that were just as bad, though in a different way, as those of an old-time institution.

As the waiting list for beds at the hospital was never less, and sometimes more, than seventy geriatrics, I was reluctant initially to go out and see old folk, because I felt that if I couldn't offer them a bed it was somehow my fault. Then I realized that even if I couldn't get them into hospital, for the moment anyway, it helped the patient to be visited – at the very least I was able to order sedation and talk to the relatives.

At first I was far more concerned about the aged who lived on their own. Far too often things got desperate for them in winter, when the weather was too bad for them to go out shopping, and they stayed in bed to economize on fuel. As bed weakened them, they tended to live on such easy-to-get meals as milk and cornflakes, and they became more weak and confused from malnutrition. The weaker they got, the more cornflakes and bread and butter became their staple diet. It was wonderful to see the way a terribly confused old lady became rational and calm after a short course of vitamin injections in hospital.

The isolation of living on their own, often without visitors because their relatives didn't bother or there weren't any, further disorientated the old people, and they became a worry to the policemen owing to their habit of wandering out at night, or, if they were lucky enough to possess telephones, phoning the police station and saying that they had been burgled. Another danger was their habit of turning up gas fires and cookers. Neighbours so often did their best to help their old folk, but they couldn't be there all the time and they felt, with some justification, that help should also come from relatives or the hospital.

Lonely though they were, many of the aged clung to familiar surroundings with heartbreaking tenacity. I remember the first old woman I was asked to visit. She lived in a small house in a dirty little terrace, and when we opened the door the smell of damp and fustiness in the house was overpowering. The patient herself was a tiny old woman with paper-thin bones and a frantically apologetic air. She cowered behind a chair in the dark little kitchen. All the warmth in the house was provided via the open oven door.

A spinster who had been a maid all her life, without relatives, had a bad heart, was on five sorts of pills prescribed by her GP and lived entirely on her own. The woman next door was tired of looking to see that she didn't wander out at night, and the police were fed up at her turning up there saying she had heard a noise on her roof. She was quite disorientated and couldn't tell me her age. She looked half-starved, and I could only see some stale-looking bread and a half-bottle of milk in the house. Her GP wanted her to come into Bushy Park. She would certainly benefit from good food and a warm bed, the MWO added.

When I mentioned hospital to the old woman she shivered, folded her arms across her scrawny chest, and begged me not to 'put her away'. I tried to explain that she could come in voluntarily, but, to her, going into a hospital like Bushy Park was the end. There were no real grounds for putting her on a certificate. Maybe she'd live longer in hospital than here amongst the dirt and the cold, but if she wanted to die in her own home, ramshackle though it was, then that was her privilege; I therefore asked the MWO to try to get her a Home Help and some Meals-on-Wheels service. But whenever I visited her after that a look of fright would come across her face, and I would have to assure her over and over that I wasn't forcing her to come into hospital.

Sometimes a husband and wife grew old together, without children or near relatives. One ancient couple I was asked to see looked physically well preserved and were obviously very devoted. The old man told me that his wife was 'going a little funny' and that he was very worried about her. She was indeed demented to some extent, but I discovered that her husband was in fact just as senile, though, being a little more intelligent, he could disguise it more easily. Both of them didn't sleep well, and for a long time shopping and cooking had been impossible due to their various disabilities. A short spell in hospital would set them up, so I suggested them coming in for two weeks.

'Us two? Would we be parted?' The old man was the first to grasp that this might happen. 'We've always been together for forty years.'

To my horror they both started to weep helplessly, and the MWO looked at me reproachfully. I quickly had to assure the old pair that I was in no position to force them to come.

A demented or senile old person can put tremendous strains on the relative or relatives who, with the best will in the world, want to look after them. One daughter of fifty had to rely on neighbours to enable her to go out shopping; unsupervised, her old mother would have fallen into the fire again, as she had done on several occasions. I took this old woman, who was quite demented, into hospital, knowing that if the daughter didn't get a rest soon, she would have a complete breakdown.

Often tensions were generated when a house accommodated different generations. Granny might decide to come downstairs in her nightgown in the middle of a young party, and disgrace her grandchildren by talking rubbish. The children of the old person often had such difficulty coping with divided loyalties that they cracked up themselves. It is a great strain having to spoon-feed an aged person, change his sheets maybe twice a night, and follow him around during the day to see that he doesn't throw off his or her clothes or have a fall.

Mr Tomkins was a deceptively spry-looking old man of seventy-five, who had been retired from his job with the Dock Board for many years. Miss Benson, a jolly young MWO, had been looking in on him since his wife died, as he only had one daughter who lived down south. Lately he had been turning up all the lights in his bungalow for most of the night, and during the day he would wander into the 'local' and stand round after round of drinks. The landlord, who was fond of the old man, said that at this rate his money would soon be gone.

'He really shouldn't be living on his own,' Miss Benson said as she drove us towards a modern bungalow in one of the residential areas of Haxton. 'But I'm sure he won't want to come into hospital. By the way, I've told him that a specialist is coming to see him. Let's hope he hasn't gone out.'

A thin man, with clear pink skin, fluffy white hair and thick glasses, answered the door to us. He wore a warm cardigan and a clean shirt, but I noticed he only had one slipper on.

'Come in. Oh, Miss Benson, you didn't tell me that the specialist would be a lady! Come in.'

He led us into a very comfortable lounge. We sat down and I began to take off layers of clothes. The gas fire must have been kept on high for ages. When Miss Benson asked him if she could lower it, he replied vaguely that she could do anything she wanted.

He'd like to offer us tea, he said, but the milkman hadn't

come. Would we care for a drink? Before we could say anything, he rushed out and reappeared with three glasses on a tray. Thinking it was lemonade, I took a fair gulp and nearly expired – it was neat gin! Miss Benson was more cautious and I followed her example by slipping my drink out of sight.

Mr Tomkins didn't notice our not drinking; his attention-span was as limited as a child's. He asked us to come and look round the bungalow, and he skipped about, opening cupboards, pulling out shelves, and leaping on the large double-bed in the bedroom to demonstrate how comfortable it was.

'You're not eating, Mr Tomkins,' Miss Benson said, looking into the empty fridge in the kitchen. 'His wife did all the cooking,' she whispered to me.

He hadn't time to eat, Mr Tomkins said absently, as he whipped out a new and very expensive heater and clicked it on, making the air more stifling than ever. 'There's so much to be done, Specialist.' He looked at me for understanding, but didn't elaborate on what he had to do.

I murmured something about his having a lovely home, and he said sharply, 'Yes, yes. And lovely it is to see you, Specialist, but *why* have you come?'

'Well,' I said, 'I think that you have been overdoing things and you need a rest.'

The word 'rest' could be used to cover a great many things. Clearly, Mr Tomkins was dangerous to himself the way he was going on, but I wanted him to come into hospital as a voluntary or 'informal' patient.

'Rest? Where?' He looked at Miss Benson as if she had brought some dangerous animal to see him.

'In Bushy Park Hospital.'

I always told the patients exactly where they were going. Too often they were told they were going to a hotel or to a *general* hospital; one poor old man was even informed that he was going to play a football match against Bushy Park! When patients discovered any deception, they often became hyper-suspicious of the staff.

'Bushy Park? Oh, Specialist!' Mr Tomkins sat down at the end of the bed, produced an enormous handkerchief, and sobbed into it. I felt dreadful coming into the poor old man's nice home and behaving like a psychiatric bailiff, but what was the alternative? Mr Tomkins would spend all his money; he wasn't looking after himself or sleeping; and his daughter was very worried about him.

Miss Benson weighed in and said that Mr Tomkins could go to the nice new unit which was up the road from the main part of the hospital. It would only be for a short time and she would see to things here at the bungalow.

Mr Tomkins wept for a long time and refused to go as an in-patient so we compromised, and I arranged for him to attend the Day Hospital. Miss Benson would fix for the ambulance to collect him every morning and leave him at home in the evenings.

I called in to the Day Unit to see Mr Tomkins three days later. Mr Canning, the nurse-in-charge, said yes, he had arrived and had settled down very well. I saw *how* well he was when he appeared in the corridor, with a ripe-looking blonde in tow.

'Hallo, Specialist,' he shouted. He looked flushed and his eyes were blazing. 'I *like* it here. It's lovely. I'm sorry I didn't come in before!'

He galloped off, hand in hand with the girl!

Unfortunately Mr Tomkins got so excitable that he had to come as an in-patient. He was more than agreeable to this, having been eased into hospital life by his attendance at the Day Unit, but on his second weekend leave he got knocked down by a car in front of his bungalow. He was dead before he reached the hospital.

The fact that I was a woman resulted in my seeing more female patients than male. The GPs tended to take the view that because of my sex their female patients would feel more at home with me. Although I really don't mind if I see only male or female patients for short periods, it would be very dull (and not good for doctor or patient) to have a one-sex clientele.

Being a woman also made child referrals more likely, especially as we didn't have a child psychiatrist in Haxton for a long time. As I had had no formal training in child psychiatry, I was very nervous about trying to treat very young people, and I often thought that the GPs were more practised at it than I was!

A case that taught me a lesson, and caused several new white hairs to appear, involved a young woman and her child. The lesson I learned in dealing with Mrs Kershaw was that never, ever, should one fail to act on the feeling that all is not well with a patient. The more I did psychiatry, the more I became conscious on some occasions of having a sort of unscientific 'hunch' that an individual was 'out of true' mentally, even though superficially he might be stable. Very often you have nothing to go on: your questions are answered blandly and correctly, and you feel like apologizing to the patient for even referring to them as such. But that patient haunts you.

Mrs Kershaw's doctor rang me up one morning and asked if I would do a 'Dom' on her; she didn't want to go to a psychiatric out-patients'. His reason for wanting advice was that Mrs Kershaw, a young mother of twenty-five, had taken a dislike to her young son and had beaten him up so badly that Mr Kershaw had taken the child to stay with his mother for a while. Dr Grant couldn't find anything very wrong with the girl, and as far as he could see the marriage was happy.

I had expected to find a tense mother whose nerves were too bad to allow her to leave the house, but the girl who answered my knock was very much in control of herself. She had a round, pretty face and longish hair, tied back with a black bow. She wore a smart red blouse and a black skirt.

The house was one of those squat little buildings that look much worse outside than indoors. The young couple must have worked hard on it; the paintwork was fresh and there was an apple-green fitted carpet. A huge TV set and radiogram stood in one corner, and there was central heating.

I wondered why Mrs Kershaw couldn't come to the clinic. She didn't give any reason, but sat quietly in a corner of the settee and said she supposed that Dr Grant had sent me.

'That's right,' I said. Then I was aware of a noise behind the chair, and a small boy of three crept out. He ran over to Mrs Kershaw, who picked him up. He sat gravely on her lap and stared over at me.

'Well,' she said, 'this is Ian. I have another son, Adrian, who's four and . . . well, ever since he was born I haven't liked him. At times I get so irritated with him that I can't control myself and I belt him. I don't *want* to hit him – I just can't help it. Something comes over me . . . it's terrible. I've *tried* to love him, but love isn't something you can turn on like a tap, is it?'

I tried to go over the possibilities. Fortunately you don't meet many Mrs Kershaws. It's common enough for a woman not to want a child and then love it when it's born; or, alternatively, it happens in many families, and amongst good mothers, that although they love all their children, they are unable to control an excess of affection for one child. And there are instances where women are cruel to their children, not so much because they don't love them but due to the pressures of lack of money, a bad husband or perhaps their own ill health, all making them unable to control their tempers.

'You can't turn it on like a tap, can you?' she repeated in a voice that was, I felt, unconsciously cold and rejecting.

There *must* be a reason for this normal-looking girl to have no feeling for her first-born. The obvious explanation was that the child wasn't her husband's, but she denied this when I put it to her and said that not only was it her husband's but that they both of them had wanted a boy, and Adrian was a handsome little boy, well-behaved, too. Yes, she was happily married; everything was all right there. Her husband earned good money and they got on well together.

I tried to find out what sort of childhood and adolescence she'd had, but I drew a blank there. She had been happy as one of a large family, and she got on well with her parents, who were still alive. She had worked as a clerk for four years before getting married.

'And how do you feel . . . in yourself?' She certainly looked like any other well-dressed young mother, and I had to keep remembering that she had beaten her eldest son very severely indeed.

'I feel all right, apart from this irritation with Adrian. I mean, Frank, that's my husband, is very fond of the lad, and he's saying that the child would be better with his Gran, that's Frank's mother.'

'Do you find that you lose your temper with other people?'

'Not to the extent that I do with Adrian. It's awful . . . he'll come up to me and try to climb into my lap and I want to push him away. I've thought and thought about it, and I don't know why I should feel this way. Frank says it's unnatural, but what can you do?'

I didn't know what to do. There was something wrong somewhere but my probing hadn't found it. I said I'd like Mrs Kershaw to come into hospital but I wasn't surprised when she refused. I asked her if she would be able to visit me at Bushy Park, if she didn't like going to an out-patients' clinic.

'I don't mind coming to see you; it's just that there's a lot round here going and I just don't want them saying I'm a nut case. Along with everything else . . .'

I said that I would see her the following week on a Wednesday morning, and I asked her to bring her husband along.

I couldn't get Mrs Kershaw out of my head the whole week, and somehow it wasn't a surprise when Mr Morgan, a kindly MWO with a face like an old boot and a tangle of black hair that he never had time to get cut, rang me up on Tuesday night.

'Sorry for disturbing you when you're not on duty, Doctor, but I thought you'd be interested. Mrs Kershaw attacked Adrian so badly that he's had to be admitted to the General Hospital with a fractured skull.'

Oh, God! I pictured a small corpse and then, almost worse, a brain-damaged little boy.

'I thought the boy was with his grandmother?'

'The husband took him home. Anyhow, we've got an immediate court order so as to remove the child from his mother.'

I castigated myself savagely. I should have pestered her more. I should have seen the father and warned him not to take the child home. I should have seen Mrs Kershaw sooner. I should have insisted upon her coming into hospital immediately . . .

Adrian got better and Mrs Kershaw did come into Bushy

Park; after having tests done it was found that she had a form of epilepsy, which was treatable.

Later, when I tried to find out whether Adrian was ever returned to her, I learnt that the Kershaws had vanished from the district.

CHAPTER THIRTEEN

The golden rule in dealing with disturbed children is, look for the faults in parental control and in the parents themselves. With the exception of the few children who are born with brain abnormalities, or who develop a mental illness after birth, disturbed children who behave in a neurotic way do so because of their parents. Ambrose Tasker would never have become the gasping, pallid child that he was if it weren't for the stifling aura generated by his monstrous parents.

It was Dr Marie Reynolds, partner in a Haxton husband-and-wife practice, who asked me to go and see Mrs Sutton, the mother of seven-year-old identical twin girls. They were over-active to such a degree that their mother was in danger of complete nervous collapse.

'And if Mother is ill, God knows what will happen to the twins,' Marie said, 'because they really are impossible to deal with. They were overactive from birth. Their mother took them to see two children's specialists, who both agreed that they were hyperkinetic but, apart from that, perfectly normal intelligent girls. The thing is that they only sleep about three hours every night, and then start racing around, waking up Mother. I've tried them on huge doses of hypnotics but they still won't sleep. It's really a worry what to do next.'

I listened to Marie Reynolds with great respect because she had five healthy children herself, although you wouldn't think it from her appearance, which was as smart as paint, and the amount of work that she did in the practice.

'I've never come across children like them,' she said. 'The parents were happy, and Mrs Sutton was a good mother. She wanted one child and, after an interval, maybe one more. She just didn't allow for Fate giving her two human bombs.'

Mrs Sutton was a petite girl, who would have been attractive if it weren't for her pallor and the way her bones jutted out. She walked into the sitting-room as if she were recovering from an illness. The twins were with her mother, she said; she was about the only person who would have them.

In between her darts to the window to see whether the children were coming back, Mrs Sutton told me about the strain of living with this tornado-like pair. The daytimes were bad enough, she said, especially when it was wet, as the little girls were never still and galloped around making a terrible noise. They wouldn't stay quiet to watch television ever, and all she could do was sit and read them stories. Because they frightened other children with their energy, she didn't take them out except for an odd walk to the park, and nobody called to see her except her mother. The nights were the worst, though; she herself used to be a normal sleeper but now she only slept when the children did. She used to go in to them when they woke, but she was too tired now to keep this up, and all she could do was lie and listen to the din as they raced around the room. Sometimes she went downstairs and made a cup of tea.

'But what about your husband, Mrs Sutton?'

'Oh, it's all right for him,' she said apathetically. 'He works so hard that he's off as soon as his head's on the pillow. No, the twins never disturb Jack.'

There was a pattering noise outside and the sound of a key being turned in the lock. Two red-cheeked girls, wearing white fur coats, burst in and rushed up to me, staring at me for a minute before racing around me.

'Never seen a pair like them,' said Gran, a mild-looking woman who looked almost as tired as Mrs Sutton.

'Brenda, that's the Doctor's coat . . . Beverley!' Mrs Sutton snatched my coat from the children, who were using it as a tent to wrestle in. They dropped it and then one of them tried to reach a bag of sweets on the table and pulled over a bottle of ink, while her twin bawled that she was thirsty and wanted a drink. Mrs Sutton had told me which was which, but they both looked exactly the same to me. Everything about them was larger than life; they were stronger than was normal for their age, their voices were piercingly loud, and I could see by their curiosity and from what they said that they were brighter than average.

'Mother, take them into the kitchen. I got a big bottle of Coke yesterday. It's behind the cupboard in the back room.'

Gran and the children trooped out, with the girls shouting 'Coke! Coke!', but Gran was back in a minute to say she couldn't find it.

'Oh, that's Beverley!' Mother declared. 'She finds everything I hide. They neither of them eat a lot, but they love drinks. Last Christmas I noticed that the level in a bottle of whisky was going down and down, and I came in one day and found Beverley in a coma. She'd been coming in every day and sipping at the whisky. I had to take her to hospital.'

'When they stayed with me,' Gran began, anxious to have her say, 'I tried giving them whisky at night to put them off, but, Lord save us, I found that half a bottle went nowhere in a night with them, so I had to stop. It's certainly not from you, dear, that they get this. You were a good little thing. I remember you going up to bed ever so quietly with your book and your doll. I used to pop in half an hour later and take the book out of your hand, and you were in such a deep sleep that you never heard me.'

'She blames Jack's family for the twins,' Mrs Sutton explained, drooping herself in a chair. She really looked as if she needed two weeks in bed. 'There were twins in his family, and he has an aunt who's a bit odd. Is there anything I can give them, Doctor? I can't go on like this, it's really getting me down. Dr Reynolds says she daren't give them any more drugs at night; they're on the highest dose that's safe.'

I said that I would write to Dr Reynolds about the twins and would order a drug that I hoped would calm them a little. I would also like to call and see the family in two weeks' time.

As the twins had had every sort of investigation and test, with negative results, there didn't seem any point in sending them to see another specialist. As with so many things like migraine, chestiness, tics and mannerisms, there is always the hope that children will 'grow out of it', and often they do, but the meantime can be very long, and it was clear that I would have Mrs Sutton as a patient if something wasn't done. Gran looked as if she'd had enough as well.

Although the Benzedrine group of drugs, used for cutting down appetite, are stimulative in adults, they have the opposite effect in hyperkinetic children, cutting down the hyperkinesis and exerting a general calming effect. I rang Marie Reynolds and asked her to try a small dose of such a drug three times a day, and if the children seemed to tolerate it we could increase it gradually. I suggested a tranquillizer for Mrs Sutton.

'Have you ever seen a pair like them?' Marie asked.

'Never,' I said. 'It must be one of the rare cases of a disturbance in children which is *not* due to the parents.'

'But there's no doubt Mrs Sutton is on the point of cracking up. I'd rather take on another five like my own than that pair. Last week Beverley swallowed her Gran's heart-pills, and before that we had Brenda throwing the key of the house down a drain.'

I couldn't wait until my next visit to see what effect the tablets were having so I called there after a week. The twins were sitting at a table, pummelling plasticine into imaginative shapes.

They *had* been better, Mrs Sutton said, and they would settle to something like painting far more easily than they used to. She herself looked more rested.

'If they can only keep it up,' Mrs Sutton said, 'I'll be able to get them into school next September.'

We increased the twins' tablets until they were on a whacking dose three times a day. Whenever I saw Marie Reynolds I asked about them, and she told me that they were all right while they were on drugs, but if they had to do without them they were as noisy and obstreperous as ever. Like diabetics, they seemed to be lacking some substance which needed continual replacement, but until research pinned down exactly what it was there was little more any of us could do.

Amongst my female referrals was an intelligent Scots girl who had been a kindergarten teacher. She was a neat dark girl and her little boy was shy but very well dressed. I noticed that her anxiety showed itself in the way she kept looking at the child, tidying his hair and wiping a tiny speck from his face.

'I know I'm overly tidy,' Mrs Flood said. 'I was always a bit like that, but since I've been married to Dick I've got worse. That's partly why I came to see you. You'll think I'm crazy, the house is as clean as anything but I go around washing, washing all day. Dick says I'll wear away the paintwork. I'm at it weekends and nights and I just can't stop. Look at my hands . . .' They were indeed red and swollen from detergent and disinfectant. 'I've been to the skin specialist, and he says it's due to all the washing and I must stop it. I've tried to and I can't. It's ridiculous, isn't it? Even though I wear rubber gloves . . .'

Joan Flood was an 'obsessional', someone who likes a place for everything and everything in its place. Under stress, the obsessional personality shows anxiety by becoming a slave to its desire for cleanliness and order, and this often takes the form of endless rituals and unnecessary cleaning. One patient told me that his morning ritual took no less than an hour and a half after he got up, and involved seeing that his bed hadn't a crease in it, that his pyjamas were folded in a certain way and that his shoes were immaculately polished.

'Isn't it ridiculous?' Mrs Flood said despairingly. 'This hand-washing is beginning to dominate my whole life.' She caught her small son's hand, which had a very small piece of jelly baby on it. 'Honestly, Dick is beginning to get fed up. It's awful for him to come home and find me washing sheets which, as he says, are clean enough anyway.'

It sounded as if Mrs Flood's washing was ruining the marriage, but I soon found out that the rocky marriage was making Mrs Flood so tense that her only outlet was an intensification of her tendency to be houseproud.

As I got her to talk about herself (which took ages, because she had the common attitude that to admit to your private worries was a sign of moral weakness) I had a fascinating insight into what it must be like to be married to a policeman. Dick was doing very well on the Force, I gathered. Mrs Flood was very lonely, not so much because all her family were in Scotland, but because her neighbours on the estate avoided her when they learnt that she was married to a policeman. 'It's terrible to go into a shop, say, and see a crowd of women gossiping. They stop as soon as they see me, and I know it's because of Dick.'

Her husband worked long and irregular hours. Much of his job involved getting information, and she knew that he had been unfaithful because he had arrived home once at three in the morning, with lipstick on his collar, and told her he'd had to go to a party in order to see someone who had 'useful information'. In the last year she had received three anonymous letters, one saying that the writer would 'get' her, and although she tried not to think about it she *did* worry that someone with a grievance against her husband would come to the house when he was out.

Dick was under strain, too, she admitted. Although he had always been hot-tempered, his rages were increasing and he was very strict with their little boy. She loved her husband, and understood his explosive feelings, if only *she* could get rid of her washing phobia and become calmer, she was sure that the marriage would be better.

I ordered her a tranquillizer and an anti-depressant, and said I would see her again in two weeks. If she had been an ordinary woman I'd have asked her to bring her husband along, but when I sounded her about this she said that Dick would be furious if he knew she had told anyone, even a doctor, and that he would 'go beserk' if he knew she had visited a psychiatrist.

In the next few months I saw three more policemen's wives and they all ran pretty well true to pattern – to such an extent that I began to wonder about the personalities of men who wanted to become policemen and detectives. Very often they were perfectionists, insisting on a high standard of conduct from their wives and children. One woman said that her husband, who was a constable, refused to speak to their son when he failed the Eleven-Plus. The wives were certainly lonely because their husbands' jobs placed such a strain on friendship, and their children, too, were avoided by other children. The cry of 'Your Dad's a copper' was a slur.

The wives were all intelligent and pathetically anxious to

excuse their husbands' often trying moods by maintaining that their jobs were difficult and demanding.

I was seeing interesting cases like this all the time now, and I often wished that I possessed some sense of scientific adventure. Instead of collecting case histories and doing background research, I merely noted similarities and differences and filed them all away in my mind. If I had been Harriet my next brilliant thesis would doubtless have been entitled 'The Policemen's Wives' Syndrome'.

CHAPTER FOURTEEN

Rosie had asked me down to her cottage in Wales and I went there full of foreboding. She was bound to be pining for the active life of the hospital, and I had visions of a somewhat pathetic woman, trying to adjust to a world in which a retired doctor had no status and was only one of the millions of people who were going to swell the geriatric problem.

I needn't have worried: Rosie looked her usual self, only much more relaxed. Far from missing the hospital, she was wishing she had retired at fifty-five.

'But the patients – what about your patients? Don't you miss them?' After all, as I told her, her patients missed *her*.

'I loved my work; in fact I enjoyed my life because I did exactly what I wanted to do, but I missed an awful lot in some ways. Like cooking . . . I'm taking cookery lessons once a week at the Tech and, you know, it's great fun. I've brushed up my bridge and I play at least once a week with these Army people that I met. And then there are always things to do at home.'

So much for my worry that Rosie would turn out to be an old bore who had nothing to talk about but her menopausal ladies. Actually, she didn't talk about patients at all, and seemed uninterested in the hospital news.

'What about a locum? You might consider doing a locum in the summer,' I suggested. Surely she wasn't going to lose touch completely with medicine.

'Look, duckie, I spent most of my life working, so now I'm

going to live a little. I don't need money, so why should I work? The trouble with you is that you're too involved in hospital life. You should get out more, meet more people.'

She had me there. Now that my son was away at school for most of the year, there was no reason why I shouldn't begin to live a little, like Rosie, but I found that I had got into such a habit of making do with survival tactics that I had lost the knack of socializing. Sometimes I did get panicky at the thought of my life slipping away without my trying to make it more interesting or exciting, but I reckoned I'd done everything I wanted to. Some things hadn't turned out right, like my marriage, but no one had forced me into that; and if no one was exactly queuing up to ask me to marry again, it didn't worry me. I knew my own insecurities made me a poor matrimonial bet.

Psychiatrists are very understanding people when you have problems; they ask no awkward questions and make elastic allowances for odd behaviour. The only one who put me in a spot was Ishraf, whose tactlessness went as far as asking Roger Ashe if England was his native country!

'Such cheek,' Roger hissed afterwards, 'from someone who's used to eating with his hands!'

I continued to be absorbed in the work at Bushy Park, and although I agreed with Rosie that I should probably take up painting or learn a language, I knew my restricted, insular life gave me security. I hadn't forgotten what it had been like after my son was born, and, remembering Scarlett O'Hara in *Gone With the Wind*, I vowed that I'd never be poor again. This determination was an active, conscious thing, but my defences against being hurt again were probably mostly subconscious. Patients couldn't hurt you so it was safe to relax with them, and although I was friendly enough with my colleagues I only saw them at work and none of them knew me very well. Whenever I revealed a new side of myself they were always surprised.

Ishraf made his *faux pas* some weeks after he had arrived. As he was a strict Muslim, he didn't like the food that was served, so he used to go into the small kitchen and annoy the maids by cooking tangy concoctions of his own. He was a generous man, and he used to offer the results of his cooking to the rest of the doctors. I rather liked his curries and pilaus, so I usually let him heap samples on my plate. He always asked Roger Ashe if he would like some, and wasn't put off by Roger telling him clearly several times that his stomach wasn't strong and that he never touched 'foreign food'.

One day when the dining-room was crowded, Ishraf came in with a steaming curried fish dish. Most of the doctors refused it (including Singh, who by now had gone all Western and even gobbled down pork), much to Ishraf's disappointment, but I allowed him to pile a spicy heap of it on my plate. During the lull in the general conversation, he looked at my hand and asked solicitously, 'You are not married?'

I noticed Singh's eyes flickering disdainfully, and Ashe looked at the ceiling. I said that I had been married but was separated now, and swiftly Hedley took over and asked whether anyone was going to a particularly good film on depression which was being shown that afternoon.

Roger waited until the others had gone and commiserated with me about Ishraf's gaffe. Of course, he said comfortingly, any man who could expose his smelly feet in the dining-room had more in common with the Missing Link, and I must remember that Ishraf really wasn't very bright. Then he plunged his long arms into the pockets of his dark suit, and said lugubriously, 'He's going to try for the Membership again, Ishraf – *not* that he has a chance. I doubt if he'd get the first MB. Anyway, you know how he goes round the hospital ferreting out hearts and other medical cases to practise on? Well, Milligan says that Matron reported Ishraf to Hedley because when he was duty doctor last visiting day, there was this man visiting who said he had a bad heart and Ishraf leapt on him to examine him. One of the other visitors, not to miss out on a bit of spontaneous treatment, announced that he had a terrible chest, and before you could say Jack Robinson, my dear, there was a proper clinic going! I gather Hedley has forbidden Ishraf to go on the wards after six. He's like a *pointer* when he sees a good case . . . positively quivers!'

I couldn't help laughing at the thought of Ishraf tearing off the visitors' clothes and subjecting them to a rigorous physical examination, although Roger added with a sniff that the Haxton people were so awfully dim that he was sure many of them wouldn't mind.

'By the way, any news of Ellison?' he asked. 'It must be ghastly having to do Madley Clinic as well as those frightful DVs.'

I was afraid to explain to Roger that I had got to like Madley Out-Patients' and was thoroughly enjoying doing Doms; it would be beyond his comprehension. Besides, I couldn't help liking the man. Because his manner either terrified or irritated people, he had no friends, and I often felt that there was a great loneliness in Roger. According to Rosie, who had met her, Norma Ashe was an even greater snob than he was, and without his brains: 'As dull as a plate of porridge, but I suppose she *is* loaded, and a title is important to Roger, even if it came from brewing hops.'

But before I could answer, Roger said with some surprise, 'Well, well, well, look who's back. Come over and see.' I went over to the window. Harriet, wearing a short fur coat over a cream trouser suit, was getting out of a sedate-looking car. A man in a dark overcoat was sitting at the wheel.

'Quite respectable.' Roger studied the disappearing car. 'I thought she only had the young and penniless in her entourage. Where did she go on holiday? And who with?'

I said I didn't know and Roger told me to be sure to find out. One of the endearing things about him was his love of scandalous snippets.

'Oh,' he said, turning back from the window, 'I meant to tell you: I have to go into hospital.'

'Nothing serious?'

'No, no. It's my tonsils. Yes, it sounds ridiculous but I've been plagued with tonsillitis, and as I don't particularly want to get resistant to antibiotics, I'm going to have them taken out by Tony Marsh.' Marsh was the ENT surgeon at the General Hospital in Haxton. 'I'm going in two weeks' time. Shouldn't be in more than a week or two.'

I was going to tell him that I would come and visit him when the door opened and Harriet came in. She had gained some weight and her face was less drawn.

'Hi, Roger . . . Hi, Joyce. Any grub left?'

She slopped some soup into a bowl, snatched a roll and came over beside us.

'Nice to see you back,' I said. 'Had a nice holiday?'

'Fantastic, really fantastic . . . I stayed with me uncle and aunt in London and I had a fabulous time. It was all go.'

Roger watched her in amazement as she lapped up her soup, dunking the roll into the liquid and gobbling the soggy pieces.

'Yeah, it was great.' She wiped her mouth with the back of her hand. 'Not one grotty day. I went to *Hair* and the new Gielgud play, and this guy I met on the train took me to the Ritz for tea. And on the way home I met this MP, and you know what he said? "Harriet, my girl, you should be in Parliament." That's what he said, "You should be in Parliament." How would you like to see me in action in the House, Rog?'

Roger said that he was sure she would be very well able to hold her own in the House, and she burst out laughing and jumped up to pour herself a cup of cold coffee.

I believed Harriet's stories of all her encounters. Her technique on the train, for instance, was to chance her arm and go into the first class compartment. She would close her eyes and pretend to be asleep, and then when the ticket collector came she would flutter her eyes and tell him she was a doctor just come off night duty, and she hadn't noticed it was a first-class compartment. If he was mean enough to pursue this, she would say helplessly that she had no money, and as she always chose a carriage with affluent-looking men in it, some dazzled gentleman would stump up for her ticket.

'God,' she groaned, 'it's so grotty being back . . . Well, what's been happening in this Nerve Centre? Has Hedley run off with a blonde and Mason put the gun to his head?'

Roger sniggered. That was just the sort of joke against Hedley and Mason's respectability that he loved. 'Oh, Ishraf is being more unbearable than ever. If he's not subjecting unfortunates to one of his endless examinations, he's in the kitchen making the maids' life hell, smoking them out with one of those petrified haggises that he calls a curry. And a coal-black man smelling of violets appeared in the wards this morning, and introduced himself as Dr Kumil, my new registrar. I think Hedley has done it deliberately, you know.'

Harriet put down her coffee cup and said that she'd had a letter that morning to say she had been awarded the MD.

'Good,' I said.

'Well done!' Roger looked at her with increased favour. He worshipped at the shrine of Intelligence as well as Good Breeding, and if Harriet failed him in the latter she certainly came up to his expectations in the former.

'Yeah, I'm delighted,' she said. 'Harry, that's the bank manager, is taking me out tonight. I see I'm on bloody duty tomorrow night.'

She looked excited, but well and back to her usual ebullient vulgarity.

At that moment a young Indian, sleek and well fed, came in and sidled up to Roger.

'I have been going round the vards, sir, and I vonder if you vould be kind enough to tell me about some of the cases? You see, I am going for my examination, vhich is in Psychiatry, in June, and so I am seeking instruction—'

Ashe turned on him furiously. 'I really haven't got the time now, Doctor. I am going on a consultation. And do try to remember that you pronounce "w" as "w", not as "v". It makes everything so confusing, like saying "She" for "He". Excuse me.'

He went out quickly, and the Indian gazed after him, puzzled.

'He is a vell-qualified man, Dr Ashe. Better than the others . . . I have looked him up. I hope that I shall get good instruction from him. Could you tell me vhere is the bank, so I can get some money, please?'

I directed him and he went out.

'Poor sod! Shame, isn't it, the way Roger takes the mickey out of them?' Harriet stuck another cigarette in her mouth. 'He can be very sadistic, Rog. Listen, Joyce, I went to a very good man in Harley Street and had him give me a really good examination, because honestly I think old Maxie is past it. He couldn't read the ECG. This bloke was twenty-five guineas but worth every penny.'

I was shocked. Had she said that she was a doctor?

'Yeah, but Harley Street is Harley Street. The thing is, I've got very bad anaemia, and he thinks that I had pleurisy and walked around with it, so no wonder I wasn't well.'

She looked me straight in the eye, as if daring me to say anything, so I didn't. And having thrown down the gauntlet, she stubbed out her cigarette and said gaily, 'I haven't heard from Tom at all, so I may as well scrub that. Did you see Harry in the car? He's terrific, really great!'

'Has he asked you to marry him?'

She jumped to her feet. 'No — but then, I don't know if I would. I mean, can you see me at coffee mornings with all the other wives? Keeping up the bourgeois image and flying the banner of respectability?'

I must say that I could not, and I didn't believe that Harry could, either.

'I don't think old Harry knows what's hit him since he met me,' she said. 'He gets shock after shock and he comes back for more. Oh well, I spent all the overdraft I had left in London. That's me lot gone.'

She drifted off, humming to herself, and I was left wondering whether she really was better. There was a curious flattening of her emotions. She appeared to voice her thoughts freely in a sort of stream-of-consciousness manner, and I remembered the fleeting reference she had made to certification and I wished that I knew her past history. She had worked in hospitals near her home town after qualification, and that's about all any of us knew. Her grandmother was dead, and this aunt and uncle were the first relatives I'd ever heard her talk about.

Later that day I came across Singh, looking darkly splendid in a brown suit with a cream shirt and tie.

'You have seen the new man, Kumil, Dr Delaney?'

'Yes, he's the new registrar, isn't he?'

'Yes. I do not like to slight one of my brethren, but really, he is just a bit better than Ishraf.' He winked at me as though we were fellow-onlookers at some Morons' Feast. 'I do not blame Ashe for getting annoyed at the manslaughter of the English language. He really is very primitive, Kumil. I say, did you see Dr Bentley since her return?'

I said I had and that she was looking very well. With some malice, I added that she had got her MD, knowing Singh had had several attempts at the MRCP.

'Yes—' he inspected his perfectly shaped nails — 'there is nothing wrong with the conative powers. It is in the emotional spheres that she is ... there is something wrong. I was at the front last night, chatting to the porter about the weather. At one in the morning there was a call to the hospital from Dr Bentley in London. She was at Euston Station, and without any money. It is a pity that she does things like that, isn't it?'

CHAPTER FIFTEEN

I met Joss Dolan the following week, and he told me that Terry Haynes came to see him regularly and that she was holding down her job. She had on several occasions been tempted to go back to prostitution and once she hadn't turned up for three weeks; but although the effort involved in keeping to the straight and narrow made her very depressed at times, she was maintaining her precarious improvement. Two old campaigners like Joss and myself knew better than to talk about patients like Terry in terms of 'cure'.

I mentioned Joan Flood, the policeman's wife, and asked Joss if he would see her.

'Sure.' He took out his little notebook. 'Give me her name and address and I'll contact her.'

I told him of my theories about policemen's wives, and said that I was pretty sure PC Flood wouldn't come along to see him, especially if he knew Joss wasn't medically qualified.

'Well, I'll *try* and get him to come.' Dolan put away his notebook, and Roger Ashe loped by, nodding his long head distantly at us.

Dolan stared after him. 'If I tried to imagine someone who shouldn't do psychiatry, Ashe would fit that category exactly. He sent me a man last week on whom he wanted an intelligence test done — which is rare, because Ashe reckons that he's the best assessor of intelligence. The man was quite shattered – Ashe had told him he was a psychopath and not a very bright one at that!'

Roger Ashe was going into hospital himself soon for a tonsillitis operation. Dolan said that he hoped the experience might give him more understanding of a patient's lot. Every time I thought about Roger's unsuitability for psychiatry, I decided that all doctors who wanted to take up mental work ought to be given a battery of tests to assess their suitability for the subject. Too often doctors either drifted into psychiatry, or deliberately chose it because it meant quicker promotion or easier working conditions. I was quite aware that I myself would fail lamentably. Like marriage, doctors often choose their speciality for all the wrong reasons.

Joss was also worried about Harriet. 'She was racing up the corridor this morning, sucking a lollipop and looking as if the furies were chasing her. Ben Williams, that's my new assistant, said that he met the nurse on one of the male admission wards where she's working and the nurse told him that they're very worried at the things she's telling patients ... All about her own private life and troubles. Is there no one who can help her? Can't any of the doctors see how ill she is?'

It was no use trying to explain to Dolan the terrible difficulties that arose when a doctor was disturbed mentally but not badly enough to make action necessary. As Harriet herself had pointed out, she wasn't certifiable.

'What if she makes a mistake in ordering a drug?' Joss asked. 'I mean, is she safe to work?'

This was the blind spot in psychologists. With all their intelligence and undoubted dedication to their work, they either were unaware of the unwritten medical codes or else didn't agree with them. Dolan saw Harriet as a doctor who wasn't functioning properly because she was ill. It seemed to him a black and white matter. To other doctors, there were many shades of grey in dealing with a mentally ill colleague. Dog didn't eat dog, hence the reluctance of other doctors to take action in a situation which they hoped would disappear if they pretended it didn't exist. To act was unpleasantly like treachery.

*   *   *

Work was the great counter-irritant, the never-failing anodyne. I went off to do the Madley Clinic with a sense of relief. The abominable weather, the smell from the knacker's yard and the dreariness of the hospital itself no longer worried me. Even the way Matron stared stonily at me, when I appeared, didn't put me out.

My first patient was a Mr Denis Wilson, who had been referred by his doctor because of increasing depression. His misery was quite apparent: dead eyes and dejected, slow movements. He was fifty, and ever since a romance had petered out ten years ago he had lived with his mother. She had died six months ago, and now he was completely on his own. He had a good job as an engineer, but he felt that he'd lost his grip completely at work. When he came home from his job he couldn't be bothered to get a meal, but sat staring at a TV set, which he wasn't interested enough even to turn on. He thought about suicide a great deal but hadn't the initiative to try it.

'And although my own doctor gives me sleeping-pills, I can't get more than about four hours' sleep, and even then I wake up at dawn.'

Mr Wilson sat in front of me, too sad for tears and past hope. There was every danger that he might just summon up enough strength to put himself out of an existence which was nothing but a miserable grind, so I asked him to come into hospital for a while. He sighed and said that the thought of going to a place like Bushy Park was intolerable: wasn't there anything else? Although I would have felt happier if he had taken my advice, I never tried to force people to come unless it was absolutely imperative. I told him therefore that I would see him every week until he was better, and that I would ask Mr Pilsworth, the Senior MWO, to call on him during the week. I was also going to write to Dr Summers, his GP, and suggest some very strong anti-depressant pills, which he would have to promise to take three times a day.

Mr Wilson said he would do anything if he didn't have to go into hospital, and in a small notebook he carefully recorded the name of the pills and the exact way he was to take them. Were there any side-effects? Should he avoid certain foods while he was taking the pills? Just how soon would they begin to work? Would his sleeping-pills interfere with the day pills?

'He's a difficult man, Wilson,' I said to Mr Pilsworth over the phone later. 'I'd much prefer him to come in to the hospital, because he really is depressed and I think there's every danger of suicide. But since he's rather obsessional, I'm sure that he will take the pills exactly as prescribed.'

'I'll keep a good eye on him, Doctor. Oh, and by the way, I looked in on the Tasker family during the week. Mr Tasker is delighted with you and says that you have a great understanding of his struggles. The whole family is down with flu, but Cedric has escaped and will be up to see you today. What a man! You've got a surprise in store, Doctor.'

Later that morning Mrs Redman came in.

'Tell me, Doctor, who *is* the young man in the gorgeous outfit waiting to see you?'

'That must be Cedric,' I said. 'He's going to London. Madley isn't his scene!'

'I should say not!' she said. 'Well, the waiting-room's full, so I'll leave you to it.'

A large young man, whose problem was impotence, kept me busy for the next three-quarters of an hour, after which I saw a middle-aged woman who gave me a very familiar refrain: *she* wasn't disturbed, it was her husband. He went out to the pub every night and came home drunk, after which he did everything he could to provoke her. The latest indignity was when he had thrown his boot at her, hitting her on the bust!

'So what I been doing,' she said, 'is slipping some of my blue tablets into his mug of tea, after he's had his supper. He goes out like a light and when he comes to he says it's too late to go out. No rows or anything . . . it's marvellous!'

I had to tell Mrs Gittings that she shouldn't give tablets prescribed for her to anybody else. Although she agreed with me, I had a feeling that she would continue to drug Mr Gittings for convenience.

Cedric sailed in next, on a breeze of delicate after-shave lotion. His outfit suited his mood, he said. He wore a strawberry-red tunic, Nehru-style, over very tight bell-bottoms. A long pink scarf floated from his neck.

'What d'you think of my red lights, Doctor?' Through his

hair he ran his slender fingers, on which a multiplicity of rings glinted.

I said that the artistically arranged streaks were very becoming and he preened. He felt a hundred per cent, he told me, and it was all due to his meeting a New Friend, who owned a very classy hairdressing salon and had done Cedric's hair for him.

'I don't know why I got myself into that state over a yobo like Anthony,' he said, tossing his magnificent head. 'Now my New Friend is *cultured*. You'd love him. He reads, oh, real *deep* stuff – and none of your pop music. Oh, no, it's *medieval* music for Ninian ... that's his name, Ninian. So I'm leaving Auntie and Uncle and going to stay with Ninian. D'you know, he's got a *soothing* personality, he really has. I haven't needed to take any tablets and I feel oh, so *well*! I don't think I really should have come. There are so many unfortunates who need your attention that I feel a *fraud* coming here. To tell you the truth, Doctor, this hospital gives me the creeps! That Matron woman stalks up and down *staring* at the patients waiting. No understanding of us *sensitive* people. Those poor patients – oh! the things they come out with, some of them. The revelations ... I don't know how you do your job. Worse than a dentist's and *no* gratitude, I suppose. Talking of which ...'

Cedric gave a huge wink and pulled out a small packet which he handed to me with a lithe bow. It was a small flagon of 'Je Reviens', and Cedric was delighted when I told him that I was very fond of the scent.

'Well, I thought the *name* was very appropriate, *not* that I want to come here again. Ah, well, I must away – I'm going out for a meal with Ninian.'

On my way home that night I remembered that I had left my library books in the hospital, so I called to collect them. As I was walking towards my car I saw the man who was in charge of the male side of the hospital, coming on duty. He was really retired, but found that he missed his job and so came back on night duty. Pat Kenny was a burly man, with very astute little blue eyes buried in a chubby snub-nosed face. He was experienced and tough when he needed to be, but he didn't forget that he had a heart, and he had a way of dealing with the most disturbed patients that was most remarkable. I had seen him pacify a spitting, aggressive, sixteen-stone male patient one night, after the patient had bitten another nurse and threatened to break a chair over anybody who went near him. When Kenny rang you up about someone at night, it was wise to get up and see the patient, because it was always some major thing that needed attention.

'Hallo, Doctor. Cold night ... Coming from Madley, are you?'

I said I was, and recalled the last night I had been on duty when a young man, sky-high from a mixture of heroin and LSD had been brought in by the police. Kenny and another nurse had gently sat with the lad and prevented him from attacking them, until the drugs wore off and he was able to talk coherently.

'We had another nice customer the other night,' Kenny said. 'Tried to murder his mother with an iron bar and then went to throw himself in the canal. Dr Bentley was on ...' He paused and looked at me from beneath his shaggy eyebrows. 'Listen, I know I shouldn't say this, Doctor, but it's about Dr Bentley. Is she ill?'

'Yes, she's not well, Mr Kenny,' I said.

'That's what I thought. But she's getting worse ... Did you know she wanders around all night? And what really worried me the other night was she said she couldn't stay in her house because it was "bugged".'

My blood chilled a bit. The fact that Harriet was deluded about her house was very sinister.

'Are you sure she said that her house was bugged, Mr Kenny?'

'Very sure. She obviously wanted to talk to someone about it. I know someone who's mentally disturbed, Doctor, after twenty-five years in the game. I'd have spent longer with her but I got called to the other end of the hospital.'

I went back to my car with the nasty feeling that now, at last, something would have to be done. I would have to see Hedley in the morning about Harriet.

CHAPTER SIXTEEN

But the next morning it was Toby Mason who came in first. With his ruddy cheeks, tweed jacket and firm stride, he looked more like a farmer on the way to buy cattle than a doctor. I always found Mason friendly enough, although his whole conversation centred around patients, a fact which infuriated Roger Ashe, who had told me quite soon after I came to Bushy Park that Mason had been a clerk in a shipping office for ten years before taking up medicine. Colourless and hard-working, he smiled a great deal, and Roger often remarked that Mason's ability to get on with people was the only reason he had been made a consultant.

Although Mason had never said anything, he must have noticed Harriet's mood, so after he'd sat down behind his desk, which was piled with toppling heaps of books, letters, journals and advertisements, I came straight to the point.

'I wanted to speak to you,' I said, 'about Harriet. Don't you think we ought to do something about her?'

He gave one of his effortless smiles, but his eyes flickered away and I realized that he wasn't going to get involved.

'Well—' he cleared his throat with a long-drawn-out rattle – 'it would seem . . . er . . . well, as if she is under some stress.'

Cowardly windbag, I thought, and I tried to force him to look at me but he wouldn't. He began to pull a dog-eared note-book out of his pocket and riffle through the pages.

'I'm very worried about her,' I went on.

He pawed at the pages of the notebook with his stubby hands, and cleared his throat again.

'I think you will find . . . er . . . that . . . er . . . something will be done at the appropriate time.'

It was incredible! 'At the appropriate time' – what a pompous, meaningless cliché. So much for his interest in psychiatry! It was a different matter when the situation involved a colleague and Mason's fat hands might be in danger of getting dirty. I gave him what I hoped was a furiously sizzling look, and went out.

I found Hedley at his desk, just putting down the telephone. He wore a blue-and-white bow tie, which didn't suit him because he was a bit too small to carry it off, but I thought of the invalid Mrs Hedley and realized that perhaps he was making a pathetic effort to keep his spirits up.

The Matron had lodged a complaint with him about Ishraf's behaviour; some relatives had written a nasty letter about being told of their brother's death too late for them to come; a student nurse had gone on the roof of the nurses' home yesterday and refused to come down for three hours – all these problems had been brought to poor Hedley, and I was sorry to be bringing him another.

'What can I do for you?' He smiled and didn't try to dodge my glance.

I waded right in and said that I was worried about Harriet, and he sighed and said that so was he. He folded his hands across his narrow chest, looking like a kindly red robin. 'It's a question of what ought to be done. She's doing her work all right, there have been no complaints about that . . .'

'But there's a great deal of gossip going on.'

'Quite. But Dr Bentley – Harriet – is the sort of girl about whom there will always be gossip, and gossip isn't enough for us to act on. Have you tried talking to her, seeing if there's anything worrying her?'

I told him about Rosie asking me to speak to Harriet, not adding anything about the drug theory, and that Harriet had been to see Maxwell Evans, who had found nothing organic the matter with her.

Hedley nodded and sighed again. 'I'll have a word with Harriet this morning and try to get her to come into one of my private beds in Hope Ward. It's always best when medical and nursing staff are suffering from breakdowns for them to go to a hospital other than their local one, but in this case I think we'll just have to get her to agree to stay in hospital for a bit and take it from there.'

I told him of Kenny's account of Harriet saying that her house was 'bugged' and he said, 'Kenny wouldn't make that up, he's very astute in sizing up people. Will you be around later this morning?'

I said I would, and he picked up the phone.

'Tell Dr Bentley I want to see her as soon as she comes in.' He put down the phone and added, 'I'll try and get her to come in today, if she agrees.'

'If she doesn't?'

'Then we're really in trouble. It's hellish when a colleague is mentally ill, especially when they're like Harriet, just hovering between complete instability and normality.'

I told him about her remark about certification, and he said no doctor would dare to put a certificate on her, even if he wanted to.

'It would be interesting to know her past history,' he said, getting up and sighing again. 'I gather there are no close relatives other than the uncle and aunt in London.'

It was only when I was halfway up the corridor that it dawned on me about Hope Ward: if Harriet went in, she would be quite near to Roger, who was still in for his tonsillectomy, because Hope was a comparatively small unit and built in one compact block.

I was having a cup of coffee with Milligan in Roger's ward when the phone went. Hedley had seen Harriet, and she had agreed to go into Hope Ward today for what was to be known to the rest of the hospital as a 'check-up'. I offered to drive her down but Dave said that she had gone to her house and that he himself would take her down, as he had a clinic at the hospital that afternoon.

'How is Dr Ashe?' Milligan had a pinkish eye-shadow that made her look as if she had been crying. 'I hear he's had his tonsils out. I hope he's not feeling "dull and stupid".'

She giggled. I knew that I should have checked her for taking what Rosie would have called 'a liberty', but I was beginning to worry about what Roger would say when he found out that Harriet was a patient in Hope.

'Oh, he was really terrible before he went away,' Milligan said. 'Must have had a sore throat or something. Look at some of the things he's written in the case notes.'

She picked up one and showed me an extract:

'Her husband wants to take her out for the weekend: God help him!'

'This patient says she is mad: how true!'

'I do not consider this woman to be mad: she is a BAD LOT!'

I thought I had better call and give Harriet a hand, and anyway, I wanted to find out what sort of mood she was in. If she found out that I had gone to Hedley, she would have every reason for calling me a mischievous nosey-parker who couldn't mind her own business. She had taken my last interference very amiably, but this was a different matter.

I needn't have worried: Harriet was in a manic mood, and if she was worried she hid it very well. She answered the door dressed in a smart aubergine suit, with her hair held back by an Alice-band to match. She was smoking.

'Hi, Joyce ... have you heard the news? I'm going into a room in Hope for a rest. I think Hedley agrees with me that Evans couldn't read the ECG properly. What did I do with me fag? God, I've left the iron on ...' There was a smell of burning, and she dashed back to where the iron was smoking on the board. 'Oh, bloody hell, me best nightgown ...'

There was nothing left but a fringe of the orange lace garment and she rushed out to throw it away.

'I'm not taking too many things. A wireless, slippers ... Come into the bedroom while I make sure I haven't forgotten something. Do you want a coffee? Just as well ... there's no milk as usual. What do you think of this?'

She picked up a very expensive flask of scent and sprayed it under my nose.

'The bank manager gave me that. I haven't seen him for ages, though. Now, let me see, what else do I want? Oh, yes, a dressing-gown.'

Harriet's bedroom was even more untidy than her sitting-room. The big bed was unmade and there was something lascivious about its rumples. There was a bottle of *vin rosé* standing on the cigarette-stained bed-table that must have been opened and forgotten. The dressing-table was littered with jars of make-up that had never been touched, and in a corner stood a black corset, straight out of a Toulouse Lautrec.

Chattering away, Harriet crammed clothes into her suitcase, and asked me whether I would bring down anything she had forgotten to the hospital.

'Now ... electricity to be turned off. You'll bring down me post, won't you? Oh, I can phone everybody from the hospital, can't I? I think I hear Dave outside. He's not a bad sod, is he? Of course, I say anything to him, you know ... Well—' she stood beside her suitcase and looked around the bedroom – 'that's it, then. If that bed could only talk! Mind you, I've not been able to get any sleep in it, not lately, anyway. Most of the nights I've sat outside, drinking coffee.'

I thought about Kenny saying that she wandered around at night.

When she opened the hall door, Hedley was standing outside. He took her suitcase politely and I shut the door. Halfway to the car, Harriet screamed that she hadn't turned off the water and had forgotten her pen, so while Hedley hovered uncertainly she rushed back into the house.

'Has she got anyone to go in and see to things while she's away?' Hedley asked.

I said 'No' and he said he'd ask Matron to get someone to go in and clean the house for her. Hedley could be very kind, I thought. Whether he would be able to deal with Harriet was another matter, but at least, unlike Mason and Ashe, he was prepared to try and help. Then Harriet flashed past me, hair flying, handbag gaping open, and together they drove off.

It didn't take long for the news to percolate. Sister Eccles was hanging round the door of her ward the same day and she made a sort of sideways dart at me.

'Dr Delaney, the very one ... Is it true about Dr Bentley? I heard something about her going into hospital . . . terrible thing. I wonder what it is? Highly strung, would you say?'

I could have done without Eccles's nervous ruminations, but behind her odd manner she was genuinely fond of Harriet, so I told her that Harriet had gone into Haxton General Hospital for a rest and a check-up.

'Oh, is that it? Ah, well ... Hmmmm ... indeed. God between us and all harm, wasn't it only two days ago I went into the office and there she was, sitting sucking a lollipop ... like a *child*. But very *good hearted* ... to the old people. You know what I mean?'

'Yes, Eccles, I know what you mean.'

I left poor Eccles contorted with embarrassment, and walked on down the corridor. Mr Cotton, the new Mental Welfare Officer, was waiting for me. We were going on a Domiciliary Visit and Mr Cotton said that it was a difficult one and had the GP phoned me about it? 'Mr Unsworth. John Unsworth.'

As we drove away, I remembered. 'This is a hellishly difficult one,' Dr Lumsden had said on the phone. 'I inherited it when I took over the practice two years ago. The thing is, John Unsworth had a spinal injury fifteen years ago, which was thoroughly investigated, but ever since then he complains of intractable pain and has been on daily doses of Morphine and Pethidine that are large enough to sink a battleship. The real bogy is Mrs Unsworth, who is a very odd woman and comes down to the surgery saying that we're doing nothing for her husband. I've tried reducing the drugs, but she kicks up a terrific fuss. My partner and I think that the husband isn't in such pain as his wife makes out. I'd be glad of your opinion.'

Dr Lumsden was right about Mrs Unsworth. She was a lean woman wrapped in a man's coat, and her eyes were dull and her voice slightly slurred. Very reluctantly she let us in, and then, huddled at the edge of a shabby chair, she launched an attack on all doctors. Nobody cared about her John: she had to fight to get his drugs, and yet who was there to help her when he was racked with pain? If it wasn't for her, what would become of her husband? She looked at the clock and, muttering that it was time for John to have his injection, opened a drawer. While Mr Cotton and I watched open-mouthed, she filled a syringe from a large bottle of the powerful pain-killer Pethidine.

'Could we see Mr Unsworth?' I asked. I was beginning to formulate a theory: Mrs Unsworth had definitely taken something herself. Could it be that *she* was the drug addict and was using her husband as bait to get the stuff?

My suspicion grew when she grudgingly allowed us to see her husband. He was a thin pale man who lay apathetically in his bed, stroking a fierce-looking black cat. When he had had his injection I asked him about his pain, and he said without expression that yes, it was bad, and the injections relieved it, but I didn't think he was telling the truth. Pain is a very subjective thing. If somebody tells you they have a bad pain it's impossible to disprove them, but after being in medicine for some time you can usually tell if someone really is in pain. There is a drawn look about the face, the nostrils are pinched and the person moves with exquisite care lest he increase his agony. Mr Unsworth was languid and monosyllabic, and he seemed like a marionette, looking every so often at his wife.

Downstairs, she said fiercely that if the doctors had real mercy they would finish her husband off and not let him lie in pain for years. When I suggested his coming into hospital for observation and to see whether we could do something for his pain, I thought she was going to strike me.

I needn't think that *she* was a sucker, she said, clutching the black cat which had sprung into her lap from nowhere. *She* knew what went on in hospitals: she had read about patients having healthy organs snatched out by hungry doctors wanting material for transplants, and her John was going to die without that sort of thing.

Vainly I remonstrated that if her husband had a brief spell in hospital it would give *her* a rest.

'Think about it,' I said. I would have liked to get Mr Unsworth in to try and assess just how much he needed the lethal drugs. It wouldn't be ethical to give him a syringe full of sterile water when he said he had pain, but it would be extremely interesting.

'I won't let him go!' Mrs Unsworth nearly spat at me. 'All these years I've nursed him, night and day, nobody knows, NOBODY. And I'm not delivering him into the hands of body-snatchers.'

I had had the odd patient, especially the old, who had asked to be reassured that if they came into hospital they wouldn't have a cardiac transplant or a kidney removed to give to somebody else; or a few old people feared that they would be put to sleep for ever, but I had never come across anybody like

Mrs Unsworth. She was too emotional, and she wasn't a stupid woman.

'What do you reckon, Doctor? It's a rum do, isn't it?' Mr Cotton asked as we drove back to Bushy Park.

'Indeed it is a rum do,' I said. 'I was just thinking that if Mrs Unsworth really wanted to do away with her husband she has every opportunity, and she couldn't be found out, not with all the drugs he is on. An overdose could easily be managed, and she knows enough about drugs by now. I think the reason she doesn't kill him is that she's on drugs herself and *he* is the source of supply.'

'Mind you, I thought she was "high" when we called. I looked around for signs of drink but there weren't any.'

'She wasn't drunk. She was drugged.'

There was nothing to be done at the moment, unless Mrs Unsworth changed her mind about her husband coming into hospital, and that was unlikely.

After having a meal I drove down to Haxton General Hospital. The Private Block was situated just at the back of the main hospital building. I parked the car and went into the office to the left of the door. Sister Mullen, a middle-aged woman with a calm, unflappable manner, was putting down the phone. Everyone knew Daisy Mullen: she had worked for twenty years in the Private Block and was both efficient and pleasant.

'Dr Bentley, has she settled down all right, Sister?'

'She's sleeping at the moment, Doctor. We had to ring Dr Hedley because she was terribly excited and wanting to go around the other patients, talking to them. Dr Hedley says she is in here for a rest, so I didn't think all that activity was good for her. And I think she rather upset Dr Ashe – she's in the next room to him, you see.'

Sister Mullen was obviously going to find her two doctor patients a bit of a trial.

'Yes, you see, Dr Ashe only had his op yesterday and he's still a bit weak, so he was resting quietly when Dr Bentley went in to him, and I think he got rather a shock, because afterwards he asked me to put the "Do Not Disturb" sign on his door.'

'I won't stay long with him, Sister,' I said.

'His room's first left on the next floor,' she called.

Roger was lying regally on some plumped pillows, with his bony hands clasped over his non-existent stomach. A book was lying open beside him but he wasn't reading. He gave a jump when he saw me and clicked on another light. His skin was very pallid and his cheekbones looked more accentuated, but his voice was as waspish as ever.

'Joyce, thank God it's you! Have you heard who's next door?'

'Harriet.'

'Everybody seems to have known except me. To think that I planned this op for *months*, choosing a time when I thought I'd get some peace and quiet, and now I have this hurricane beside me. It's too bad, it really is . . .'

He pulled himself up and I could see he was wearing pale-blue silk pyjamas. After sipping some thick white liquid from a small glass, he flopped back on his pillows and rubbed his face with his hands.

'She came in here jabbering away about an ECG or something, and asking me to question her in case her memory is going. Then she began to tell me that she'd read my case notes and didn't agree with some of the things in them. She ate a pound of grapes and said how nice it was that we'd be company for each other. Dear God! I know the girl is ill, but it's the *brain*, not the body, so why bring her in here? She'll wreck the place! The staff won't be able to stand her. D'you know, I've had indigestion since her visit and that's why I'm taking this antacid. *Why* did I have to pick the week she chose to go berserk? Oh, God! There's only one hope – that the drugs she's on will knock her out!'

CHAPTER SEVENTEEN

I didn't see anyone very much next morning, because I was called up to a ward to deal with little Leah Eteng, who had gone on hunger strike and hadn't eaten for four days.

Leah was an Ibo girl, who had come to England to do nursing but had never been able to complete her training because of a breakdown. When she first came to Bushy Park she sat curled up in a chair all day, looking like Topsy and muttering to herself in her own language. If any of us spoke to her, she replied in a very dignified pidgin English. She seemed to be both deluded and hallucinated and at times shouted loudly to the voices that were tormenting her. After a course of drugs she became less withdrawn and quite gay, although she never seemed to have more initiative than to do her frizzy corkscrew hair, wash herself and read the Bible. Any attempt to ask her about Africa met with no response: it may have been that she was afraid of going back. Roger said that her own tribe would tie her to a stake and leave her to die if she went back.

Periodically she went on long hunger strikes, when she refused all food and drink. Although we suspected that she had a secret store of biscuits, as the days went by she became like a shrivelled little monkey; her shiny black skin grew grey and her small face was like a death's head. She was in bed when I got to the ward and her arms looked like brittle sticks outside the bedclothes.

'Come on, Leah. It's Doctor Delaney. Now why don't you eat?'

She opened first one eye and then the other.

'It is my own desire that I do not eat. The consumption of food is my private business.'

She had on a vast bra that must have been made for a woman with a forty-inch bust. Leah's small breasts looked ridiculous.

'It's *our* business if you die, Leah, and you *will* die if you don't eat. I have told you before that you'll have to have Electric Treatment if you don't eat.'

'Not the box!' Leah gave a shriek like a train-whistle, and two nurses rushed to hold down her threshing limbs. 'I shall not permit it that you do me like that. What are you doing to me, putting shocks through my brain? It is a liberty. AAAAhhh . .' Leah gave a particularly dramatic scream.

I told her that she was only four stone eight and she couldn't go on like this and that she would have to have the treatment.

I hated giving ECT to patients who were unwilling, because apart from a distaste for treating people against their will, it has been my experience that if someone actively dreads and is frightened of some treatment, then that therapy is unlikely to make them better. But there didn't seem any choice with Leah. We had tried persuasion, coaxing, drugs, had offered her any sort of food she fancied but nothing did any good, and although before this she had broken her fast eventually, this one was lasting longer: daily she seemed to be getting more frail, and I had a horrid vision of her disappearing like a puff of grey smoke.

'Set the box up tomorrow, Sister,' I said. 'Maybe we won't have to give it.'

When I went on the ward next morning I was hoping that Leah would have eaten, but Sister told me that she had never been left alone and had eaten or drunk nothing since I saw her last.

The box was ready and waiting on the trolley outside Leah's room, and when Sister and another nurse wheeled it in, Leah shot up in bed and shouted, 'What are you doing? You are not a nice lady, Doctor Delaney. You are very cruel indeed!'

The box was plugged in and I filled a syringe with Pentothal, which is an anaesthetic, and Scoline, which is a muscle relaxant. Singh appeared and began to dip the headpieces of the box into some saline, and two nurses tried to hold down the struggling Leah, who was bellowing with such force that you wondered how such a loud sound came from such a small body.

'You are not kind, you are cruel! This is not what it says in the Bible ... Aaahh ...' Leah's voice gurgled to a halt as the Pentothal took effect and she became unconscious.

'Now.' I signalled to Singh, who carefully put down the headpieces on Leah's fuzzy head and pressed the button. We all waited for the slight shiver that indicated the electric current was passing through, but nothing happened. Singh pressed again ... and again. Still nothing. Sister inspected the plugs and said everything was OK.

'I'll turn up the voltage.' Singh twiddled with the knobs, still nothing. 'This has never happened before,' he said. 'And this ECT box is new.'

'She must have put a jinx on it,' Sister said when I told them to put the box away, because Leah was stirring and about to come round.

When she woke up a few minutes later, she looked much brighter and promptly called for eleven pieces of toast, which she gobbled voraciously. She never mentioned the ECT. Singh told me at lunch that she must have used black magic or ju-ju. Whatever it was, the treatment seemed to have been a spectacular success.

The wireless was on in Harriet's room and the bed looked as if someone had been lying on top of it, not in it. Next door I found Harriet sitting beside Roger, who was having oxygen through a mask. He looked ghastly and his face was pinched and sunken. Harriet was dressed in a bright green cat suit, with her hair tumbling down her face, and when she spoke her voice was thick.

'Poor old Rog,' she said. 'What a fright he gave us this morning. Hear what happened? Dear God! Well, I don't know what the hell drugs Hedley has me on, but I thought I was passing out. Everything was going round. Anyhow, I stumbled in to Rog in me nightgown, because I couldn't get a nurse. *He* must have thought I was very ill because he got up out of bed to help me, and the next thing he'd jack-knifed on the floor. "Come on, Harriet girl," I said to myself, "it's a cardiac arrest or a pulmonary embolus", so I gave him cardiac massage and helped him to breathe until the nurse came. Innes rushed in but he hadn't a clue, so they called Dr Pine, the chest bloke, and right enough, part of Roger's lung had collapsed. Good job I came in . . .'

'Sorry about this, Roger,' I said. He flapped one hand feebly. He looked grey and frightened, and I tried to imagine how terrifying it must feel to have part of your lungs fold up on you. Like drowning in your own secretions. Cold surgery had the reputation of being dangerous and certainly Ashe seemed to be getting more than his share. I didn't know whether to think Harriet's presence was a hindrance or a help. Certainly she always remained cool in an emergency, and I had no doubt that she did her best to help him to breathe, but would he have got the lung collapse if she hadn't given him a fright and forced him to get up out of bed?

Sister Mullen came in and clicked her tongue. 'Your supper is in the next room, Dr Bentley. Really, Dr Ashe is *not* supposed to have visitors, even medical ones!'

Mullen's normally calm air was ruffled and she gave Harriet an exasperated glance. Like many nurses and doctors in general hospitals, she believed a case like Harriet's was just an example of a tiresome girl who was having too much attention paid to her, when she could have helped herself by exerting moral pressure and taking a good pull at herself. There was too much work for the staff to have to bother about Harriet's extravagances; by comparison with the very ill patients they had to deal with, she seemed a fraud. They couldn't understand why she was taking up a room and why Dr Hedley bothered with her.

Sister bent over Roger and I followed Harriet to her room. She lifted the silver dish covers from her supper tray and then slammed them down and lit a cigarette. She lay back on the cover of her bed.

'I'm fed up, Joyce . . . And those drugs that Dave has me on, God, they make me feel so doped. Look at me mouth, all dry . . .'

Her lips were cracked, and she must have had pretty hefty doses because her voice was slurred.

'How are you sleeping?' I asked.

She had to admit that that was better, and she was sleeping eight hours a night now. As she was saying this, she yawned heavily, and a young nurse came in with two tablets and a glass of water. Harriet made a face and swallowed the tablets.

'I can't keep awake. And when I do wake up, I'm bloody bored. Dave came in this morning and I asked him how long I was going to stay in here, and he said he didn't know. He's a kind soul, but very limited. Anyway, he's got too much to do with the hospital and that invalid wife. Oh, the bank manager sent a Get Well card.' She pointed to a large and ornate card on the table by her bed. 'And I've had heaps of messages and phone calls. I don't know who told Tom, because he sent me a nice letter telling me to take a good rest. You know, there's a lot more to Rog than you think, Joyce. D'you know, I thought he was going to die when he collapsed, and he was as calm as anything. He's got guts all right. Anyway, it's nice for him that I'm beside him and can pop in and out to him and keep an eye on him.'

Harriet chattered on and seemed delighted when a crowd of nurses from the hospital came in. Although I knew she had asked Hedley what was the matter with her and how long he thought she would be in, she had a queer indifference, and I got the impression that at bottom she knew that she wasn't fit to leave hospital and didn't really care about going home.

Hedley came into lunch the following day. I waited until the others had gone and said that I was sorry to hear about Ashe.

'Very bad luck,' he agreed. 'And to think that he'd planned it all so carefully. 'Course, he's never been very strong, Roger.'

I mentioned that I had seen Harriet and he told me that they'd had a terrible two days with her. Although she was sleeping very well now, he had tried several different sorts of drugs and they seemed to do little to allay the daytime restlessness and the hyper-activity.

'She's annoying the nursing staff by going in to other patients and talking to them. Oh, they *like* her all right, don't think that, but they don't understand just how ill she is, and of course as she looks well physically, they think she's putting things on.'

'What's the diagnosis, do you think?'

'A bit of a mystery. I checked up about any previous breakdowns and she's had two pretty bad ones in the last three years. Both were hushed up, and it was put out that she was physically ill. What the hell she took up psychiatry for ... Of course, she's bright and still has some insight, which makes her very difficult to deal with. She threatens that she's going to discharge herself, and she knows damn well we can't put her on a section. I don't think that she's schizophrenic, I'd be inclined to think that she's manic depressive psychosis: that would explain the mood swings and the mania at the moment.'

I pointed out that manic depressive psychosis meant clear-cut moods of elation alternating with depression, with periods of complete lucidity in between, but Hedley answered, 'Oh, it can be atypical, you know. Besides, there's a bad family history.'

If it hadn't been apparent that Harriet really wasn't getting any better, I would have been amused by the pair of them, Harriet and Roger, during that week. Roger was euphoric to have escaped death, and Harriet was flattered to be thought well of, as she was now, by someone as intelligent and from such a background as Roger; the morning when she had come into his room and helped to rally him had created a sort of bond between them. More often than not when I went down she would be in his room, perched on the end of his bed or lying on a chair, smoking and talking.

'I think we've all underestimated Harriet,' Roger said to me one afternoon. He was in his dressing-gown, as he was now allowed up. 'There's a curious sort of innocence about her in spite of all the randy talk, and she's got a first-class brain. What she lacks is education.'

It was all rather like Pygmalion, with Roger enacting the part of Professor Higgins. Under his tuition, Harriet began to read Philosophy and History, and sometimes when I went down I would find her taking instruction from him and submitting meekly to his corrections.

But when I saw him alone, Roger had to admit that he didn't think Harriet's mental state was a great deal better. She was more rested, but her flow of thinking and the rate of her talk was as abnormal as ever.

'She'll miss me, poor kid. I go home tomorrow. Mind you, I don't mind telling you that I'll miss *her*. Made me feel young again . . . I wonder what's going to become of her?'

The nursing staff didn't share Roger's fondness for Harriet, and Mullen called me aside when I came down from Roger that night to say they had asked Dr Hedley to speak to Harriet again, because she continued to spend her time talking to the other patients. Mullen didn't approve of the time she spent with Dr Ashe, either. And did I know that Other Men had come to see Harriet? There was one awful occasion (Mullen lowered her voice and looked over her shoulder) when a young nurse had knocked and gone into Dr Bentley's room and found her in a very compromising position with one of her male visitors. It was all most irregular. Mullen was prepared to put up with people in pain, with haemorrhages, and with drips, but she didn't know where she was with Harriet, or how to deal with the girl.

'After all, she *is* a doctor,' she said. 'Although all of us wonder just *how* she can treat patients. We've never come across a doctor like her. It's a good thing Mrs Ashe doesn't mind coming in and finding her husband talking to some girl wearing a very revealing nightdress!'

The strange part of it was that Mrs Ashe, who was a mousy-looking little woman with a pleasant smile and none of Roger's acidity, seemed to like Harriet, and told me she was most grateful to her for keeping Roger amused. She didn't appear to be shocked by the girl's vulgarity; she felt very sorry for her and was going to invite her to stay for a weekend, when Harriet was out of hospital.

I guessed that Harriet and Ashe would provide enough gossip-fodder at Haxton General for many a long day.

CHAPTER EIGHTEEN

Working in a hospital, one finds one's days pretty well mapped out. As with life on board ship, time has a habit of sliding by imperceptibly, and I got a shock when I realized that I had been at Bushy Park for over a year. What had I gained? A little more money and a lot more experience, but the latter didn't count for much these days and Bushy Park was not a good springboard if you wanted promotion. There are hospitals where even the lowliest post bestows an imprimatur of quality; and there are very bad hospitals which, even if you have only had the misfortune to work there for a short period, imme-diately stamp you as suspect and set people looking up your past, making sure you are on the Medical Register and scrutinizing your references.

There were many better hospitals than Bushy Park, but there were also many worse ones, and since there was little point in moving unless for monetary or professional gain I decided to stay. At forty you have indicated your rung on the medical ladder, and all that is required is to move sideways with some dignity to let the young and energetic get past. If your ego is bruised in the scuffling, then all you have left is some dignity and the knowledge that you have had your chances, which won't come again, and there is no point in wailing about the lost years. From thirty to forty is the vital time in promoting your medical career, and I had quite deliberately spent those years in giving as much time as possible to my son, and choosing jobs not for advancement but for how much time off they would give me. I should have got myself sent off or 'seconded' to various other hospitals and units, taken more post-graduate examinations and courses, and, infinitely important, made my face familiar in the right quarters. Most heinous of all crimes in the promotion game, I had not taken care to shut my mouth but always exercised my democratic right of free speech. When I had had a bad day in the hospital and I was feeling my age, I grew very paranoid and indulged in bitter ruminations about my failure to advance myself professionally. But when I became more detached I had to admit, as I watched the young registrars dashing off to complete their training and make themselves into that most difficult of all beings, the intelligent sycophant, that you can't have everything: if I had my life all over again I'd do the same, choosing failure and adventure rather than success and dullness.

Racially, too, I wasn't enamoured of reaching the top: there was still far too much of the Celtic 'Sure, what does it matter? Won't we all go the same way?' about my outlook, and mentally I was always throwing pinches of salt to the malignant fates. It was too easy to say to myself that everything would have been different if I had had guidance in my early career, if I hadn't made a disastrous marriage, if I hadn't had to bring up a child on my own. I had been brought up to believe that apart from the poor unfortunates who were struck down with some awful disease, you get what you deserve out of life, and the best thing to do is to make your own bed as comfortable and warm as possible, because on that you have to lie.

I think a great deal of the concern I felt for Harriet arose from the sympathy I felt for another failure. She had only made it professionally because she was clever and now, with savage irony, the very functions which were her passport to some sort of security and respectability were being taken away from her. She must have realized this herself: that was why she was always asking people like Roger to test her memory, and why she idolized Intelligence. I heard her say once that she couldn't marry a stupid man, no matter how much money he had, in case she had stupid children.

After Roger had gone home she got more restless than ever, but when Hedley told me that he was going to have to give her ECT 'as a last resort', I was appalled.

'Nothing seems to touch her very much,' he said. 'I've tried everything now, and in massive doses. Did she tell you that Professor Randle came down to see her?'

'No.'

'Well, I thought I'd like another opinion before suggesting ECT. Randle agrees that what she's suffering from is more like manic depressive psychosis, rather than schizophrenia. He spent a long time with her and I think she liked him . . .'

Of course she would. Harriet had a great reverence for anyone in the academic world.

'Anyway, the Professor said that ECT was the only thing left.'

I funked going down to see Harriet before she had ECT and was glad that a wave of sickness amongst the medical staff kept us all very busy. Although people still asked about her, the gossip and conjecture had died down a lot. But those of the nursing staff who had been to see her still couldn't get over the fact that a doctor, and a clever one, should become so disturbed.

I went down to see Harriet after she had had two ECTs and found that she had gone out to the cinema.

'She's much better since that treatment, Electro-whatever-they-call-it,' Sister Mullen said. 'Much more composed. Although we all like her, nothing personal, I don't mind telling you, Doctor, it will be a tremendous relief all round when she's discharged. You see, you can't keep her in bed, can you? So she gets bored and seems to need people to talk to all the time. It's pathetic, and we're all very sorry for her, but our nursing staff just haven't the time for that sort of thing. And because she's a doctor, it makes it all the more awkward. The young nurses don't like to tell her visitors to go, and last week we found a lot of bottles in her room. She's not supposed to drink while she's on those powerful drugs, is she?'

Sister Mullen shook her head. The unit would never be quite the same after Harriet.

Although Sister had said she had many visitors, when it came down to it they were mostly young nurses who were dazzled by Harriet's verbal ability and didn't realize how ill she was. Mason hadn't called to see her; Ashe was away; and Singh had paid one visit to satisfy his curiosity. The bank manager had baled out after sending his Get Well card.

'Well, people are *afraid* of mental illness still,' said Rosie when I saw her down at the cottage that weekend. 'It's not so much that they don't want to help but they don't know how to. A mad lay person is bad enough – but a doctor – it's too much for most people, even other doctors. Is she going back to that empty house when she's discharged?'

'I think so.'

'She'll relapse. Send her down here for a few weeks when she gets out of hospital.'

I promised Rosie that I would tell Harriet of her invitation, and on the following Monday I went down to Hope.

Harriet was sitting in her room, wearing a pink polo-necked jumper and skirt. She had her eyes closed but she opened them when I went in.

'Hallo. Sit down, Joyce.' She spoke quietly and without any of her usual bounce. When she got up to switch on the big lamp, I took a good look at her. She was pale, much paler than I had ever seen her, and there was a change in her eyes: whereas before they had been blazing, they were now dead and expressionless.

'Well . . . how are you, Harriet?'

She lay back quietly on the chair again. I noticed when she reached for her cigarettes that her movements were torpid. Had Hedley increased the drugs, or was this an after-effect of ECT? Was she moving into a depressive phase of her illness? Although I was glad that she wasn't so agitated, I didn't like her abnormal slowness. This subdued and mouse-like creature wasn't Harriet. She was like a watch that had lost its spring.

'Oh, better . . . much better. I'm on ECT, you know, so I can't remember much about coming in here, but I've been thinking about before my admission here. I was very ill, wasn't I?'

I nodded, and she pulled on her cigarette silently. What had happened to her flow of talk, the giggling and the ability to demolish any unpleasant or worrying topic? To cheer her up and to reassure myself, I said that Rosie was asking for her and wanted her to go and stay at the cottage when she came out of hospital.

'Yes, I know. She wrote to me. I would like to go and stay with her.'

Harriet drew out a letter from her bag and tapped it listlessly. It took a great deal of effort for Rosie to write, as Harriet well knew, and I would have expected her to be much more excited about it. The old Harriet would have been elated, and boisterously pleased about the invitation.

'Do you miss Roger, Harriet?' We had sat in silence for several minutes, and incredibly I found myself searching for something to say. Before, it had always been difficult to get a word in with Harriet.

'Roger? Oh, yes . . . I suppose he's glad to be home, though,' she said apathetically.

'It won't be long till you're at home now, Harriet.' I sounded falsely cheerful.

'Did Hedley tell you I'm having ECT?'

'Yes, he did.'

'Yes, I'm having ECT.'

She had forgotten she had told me before.

'I sleep very well, and I am eating. I have put on four pounds.'

140

Silence again, and she stared down at the hands clasped in her lap. I searched desperately for something bright and funny to say to her. She hadn't smiled once since I had come in, just parted her lips in a listlessly polite manner. When I left, she didn't ask me when I was coming again.

I met Sister Mullen in the corridor. She was carrying a tray with Harriet's night medication on it. Didn't I see a change in Dr Bentley? she asked me. She was much more composed and calm now.

I said that that was true, and went home feeling depressed. I knew now what Harriet reminded me of – I hadn't been able to think of it while I was with her: she resembled patients who had brain operations. Leucotomy, which was done on patients in the old days when their agitation failed to respond to drugs, had sometimes resulted in their becoming sluggish as neutered cats.

'It's early days,' said Hedley defensively, when I tackled him the next day about Harriet. 'It may well be a natural down-swing after she's been "high" for so long, you know. Anyway, she's only going to have two more ECTs, and then I'm discharging her. Her aunt from London, a Mrs Roland, is coming to stay with her, but before that Harriet tells me that she's going down to stay with Rosie for a spell.'

When Roger came back to work a few days later, he told me that he had been in to see Harriet, and she had been withdrawn and listless.

'I just don't know,' he said. 'She tells me she's returning to work after coming back from Rosie's, but I agree with you: she's rather like a robot. Not that I'd like her to be tearing around the way she was, but the pendulum has swung a bit too much the other way.'

Roger had returned to his usual self. He said that while he was grateful to Harriet for being kind to him during his stay in hospital, and that her high spirits had helped him to pass the time, in retrospect he'd have settled for less drama and more peace. It had been quite a strain having her dashing in and out of his room, introducing him to her visitors and asking his opinions on everything, from whether he thought she had a double chin to sounding her knowledge of statistics.

'And her visitors,' Roger said. 'I don't know *where* she got them – young men without "H's", and women dressed in Crimplene and with Haxton accents. I hadn't anything in common with any of them. And her clothes . . . well, it's a good job that Norma, my wife, is broad-minded, because Harriet would prance into my room in sheer night attire, looking like someone who'd escaped from the Bal Tabarin. It's all very sad . . . I really don't know what's to become of the girl. Even if she pulls out of this, what's the prognosis? And of course, she should *never* marry and have children. It would be quite criminal to pass on her genes, wouldn't it? Oh, God, look what's coming. D'you know . . .'

He lowered his voice as Dr Kumil approached us, ramrod stiff in his dark suit and high white collar.

'D'you know that he creeps into the office when I'm seeing patients and *sniffs* behind me? I think it must be a nervous tic or something. There's only one thing about him: he's *slightly* better than Ishraf.'

Roger dived down a passage leading to the laboratory, and poor Kumil looked puzzled. Dr Ashe had been away and there was so much that he wanted to ask him about, but he couldn't find him to have a good talk.

'Perhaps Dr Ashe isn't all that well,' I said, feeling rather sorry for Kumil, who worked quite hard and couldn't seem to help his sniffing.

'Excuse me,' he said to me, 'I have a problem and I do not know what is the best course in dealing with it, namely, a patient Coralie Mee, who is awfully agitated and hitting out. I have tried some sedative but it is not having the desired effect. I was going to ask Dr Ashe what is the drug of choice to quieten the lady, but as you can see he is gone and . . .'

'I'll go and see Coralie, I know her,' I said.

Coralie Mee was a fat young West Indian woman, who was very schizophrenic and subject to fits when she would run up and down the ward, slamming doors and attacking anyone in her way.

When I got up to Hammond Ward, which was always kept locked because it contained very difficult female patients, most of them dangerous, I found four nurses holding Coralie down.

'She stuffed a huge piece of plaster up her nose.' The nurse nodded her head at an enormous lump of white stuff on the floor.

'She went for me with a fork and just missed my eye,' another nurse panted.

I didn't examine Coralie after her sharp white teeth had sunk agonizingly into my arm. Sister rushed off to get an injection of a tranquillizing drug, and I went to wash my wound.

'Coralie was brought back from weekend leave after she had kicked the crutches from under her father,' Sister said. 'Even Mrs Mee had to admit defeat, and you know what she's like. Last week she gave me two dark bananas and told me to save them for Coralie and take good care of them "because you know what the staff are like". Go away, Jennifer.'

Jennifer Elkins was a psychopath who had been on drugs when she was training to be a nurse, and who had perfected every attention-seeking ploy in order to get them. Before coming to us, she had cut herself almost to the bone and then gone to Casualty in Haxton General and demanded Pethidine. She had a very white face and cold blue eyes, and she was intelligent and manipulative.

'Hallo, Dr Delaney. How is Dr Bentley? Is she better from her breakdown?'

'Go back to your tea and don't be so rude!' Poor Sister got red and shooed the girl away.

The nursing staff knew all about Harriet, and it was too much to hope that it could be kept from the patients, especially the bright ones like Jennifer. But there was an element of gloating in her voice that made my blood run cold. Harriet's distress was affecting us all in a greater or lesser degree. Somehow, sometime, it would have to be resolved.

CHAPTER NINETEEN

'I hear that Dr Bentley has come out of hospital and is re-
cuperating with Dr Sanders.' Singh was always first with the
news, and we thought that this was due to his being on
friendly terms with one of the hospital telephonists, who was
celebrating her divorce. She was excellent at her job, and we
didn't mind her listening to our phone calls because that was
an occupational hazard in hospitals, but she couldn't hold her
tongue about what she heard, and so you always had to speak
in a sort of code if you made or received any calls at the hospital which might be open to gossip.

Roger looked at Singh and then changed the conversation
to the weather.

'I wasn't going to let the side down by talking to that arro-
gant Indian about a white person who is not well,' he said to
me afterwards, as we walked up the corridor together. Nothing would change Roger's implacable hatred of Indians and
other coloured people. Indeed he had managed to get rid of
Dr Kumil and have him replaced by a new Italian registrar
called Dr Rossi, who I thought was fat, greedy and lazy. Roger
assured me, however, that Rossi was really a sensitive, shy
man, appalled by the crudities of Haxton after Florence, his
native city.

Hedley was opening the office, which was always kept
locked, so while Roger went on, I stopped and asked Dave how
Harriet was.

'So-so,' he said. 'She's back on duty.'

'But I thought she was going down to Rosie?'

'She said she'd go later and that she wanted to return to
work. Oh, I don't think she's fit, but you know Harriet. I've
tried to make her duties as easy as possible, and only given her
a few wards to do.'

I looked away as he was overcome by a ferocious attack of
sneezing. A secretary came up to say that the nurses were
waiting for him in the Training School, and that a patient had

phoned, leaving his name and telephone number, to say that he felt like taking an overdose of his tablets. Hedley blew his nose, told the secretary to phone the school to say he'd be late, and asked her to get the patient's telephone number.

'And Mrs Hedley rang to remind you to call for your daughter at the party on your way home,' I heard the secretary say as Hedley went off with her.

Just then Mason passed me, walking with his head down. He hadn't gone to see Harriet, and since I mentioned that I was worried about her he'd never spoken her name. It seemed to me a dereliction of duty. He probably rationalized things to himself by feeling that the kindest thing was to ignore Harriet and yet, if she had been a patient of his, and she had been more disturbed than many of the patients he saw, would he have felt the same? Roger told me that my mistake was in thinking Mason *had* any feelings.

'He skates over the surface of things and doesn't worry,' Roger said. 'That's his forte.'

I went on to see a young man who had been brought in the night before, bruised, beaten up and incoherent after taking a mixture of drugs which included heroin. Bushy Park didn't have an Addiction Unit, although one was badly needed, and so we had to deal with the ever-increasing number of drug addicts without any special part of the hospital in which to put them.

I found the young people who were on drugs very difficult to deal with. Many of them spoke a different language, so there was semantic difficulty for a start; and the vast majority didn't see anything wrong in taking drugs and had no intention of giving them up. As a result the function of the hospital seemed to consist of 'drying out' the young addicts, replacing the nourishment and vitamins that their addiction had interfered with, and then watching helplessly as they discharged themselves to start all over again. Even before they left hospital most of them began drugging again. A large hospital is one of the easiest places to obtain drugs, for patients can hoard the tablets prescribed for them and sell them to addicts. There was always a thriving drug market in Bushy Park, which try as we would we couldn't stamp out.

Robert Dobson, the patient who had come in last night under the influence of drugs, looked pale and wan in his striped hospital nightgown. He had tow-coloured hair, which was long and flopped over his face, making him look younger than his nineteen years. He gave an enormous yawn, a sign of drug withdrawal.

I looked at the notes: Art student at Haxton College of Art; parents both working; no brothers or sisters; childhood happy; always good at school, eight 'O' levels and three 'A's.

'When did you start taking drugs, Mr Dobson?' I asked.

'When I went to Art School. Listen, when can I go home? I didn't know this was a mental hospital!'

'Do you remember the way you felt last night?' Singh's clear script in the notes said that Dobson had been very confused, so agitated that he had needed three nurses to hold him down, and continually shouting that he had been castrated.

'Not really.' The patient yawned again, and when he put one thin arm to his mouth I thought I could see the injection marks.

'You took some drugs last night?'

'Yeah . . . I went on a bad trip though.'

'How do you mean?'

'Like I mixed them . . . and some of the stuff was bad.'

I asked him what he had taken last night and he told me LSD and some heroin. Did he know that people could go permanently mad from taking LSD or having what he called 'a bad trip'? Wearily he moistened his dry swollen lips and said yes, he knew that.

'Then why take drugs? Who do you get drugs from outside?'

Hopeless to ask that one, I knew. If he told me, he might get beaten up by the 'pusher' or members of the drug ring.

'Listen, do you intend taking drugs again when you go?'

'I could say I'm going to try and kick them, couldn't I? Kid you along that I'm going to be a good boy? Listen, I can't live without drugs, just like some alchies can't live without booze. So they're going to shorten my life – *so what*? It's not much of a bloody life anyway, from what I can make of it. Anyway, we're all going to be blown up soon. When can I go? You can't keep me here!'

'You can go any time,' I said hopelessly. He was sane, intelligent and he knew the law, that we had absolutely no grounds for detaining him. He probably shouldn't have been brought to us last night. As he pulled his dressing-gown over his hollow chest and shuffled out, I was overcome with a giant wave of despair. Very soon he would be injecting drugs into his veins, 'main-lining', if he wasn't doing that already, and then it was only months until his starved and poisoned young body gave up the fight. There was some tiny satisfaction in dealing with an addict who was trying to fight his addiction and wanting to be cured, but Dobson . . . I was almost glad when the nurse asked me to see a very mad patient called Jimmy Cheesman, who had swallowed a bottle of bleach. At least I could do something for Jimmy.

I called to see Harriet that night. When I rang her doorbell, an apologetic little woman with a Cockney accent answered my ring. She introduced herself as Auntie Madge, showed me into the sitting-room and went off to make some tea.

'Hallo, Harriet,' I said. She was sitting with her back very straight in a chair, staring down at her folded hands.

'Hallo.'

I sat down on the settee and was relieved to see her take out her cigarettes.

'You were back at work today, I hear?'

She put down her packet of cigarettes and looked at me. There was no light in her eyes and her voice was toneless. I remembered a phrase Viney had used once about a patient: 'He was so low he *smelt* of depression'.

'Yes, I went to some wards. I looked at the patients for a long time, especially one woman of about forty who was sitting on her own. Another patient came up and snatched her bag and she never even noticed. You could have jabbed her with a needle and I don't believe she would have done anything. The nurse said she'd come in ten years ago and they'd tried everything . . . every drug, every treatment. She'd had visitors who used to come, but they stopped and now nobody comes near her. I couldn't stop looking at her because I saw myself . . .'

She pulled at her cigarette, and I said that that was silly, to give herself time; after all, she'd been very ill and the ECT was bound to make her feel a bit low.

'I don't feel better . . . I just feel different. Dave's done his best, but what can he do, really? The intervals between these bouts are getting shorter, you know . . .'

When Auntie Madge came in with tea and biscuits, I hoped that she would sit down with us and perhaps the talk would be easier, but after pouring out two cups of tea and trying to tempt Harriet unsuccessfully to a biscuit, she crept out.

'Auntie Madge is my father's sister. She didn't know what to make of me before, so you can imagine how scared of me she is now.'

'Why don't you go down to Rosie for the weekend?'

'I haven't the energy to pretend,' she said, stirring her tea. 'It's an effort to smile . . . to speak . . . No, don't go yet.'

I sat down again and looked helplessly at her. Only the long hair and face remained of the Harriet I knew, and even her face looked shrunken and older. If only I could give her some crumb of hope or comfort, but she understood too much, and because of that no reassurance was possible. Nobody knew why she had breakdowns of such severity and therefore nobody could help her despair.

'I can't marry . . . that's out. It wouldn't be fair to have children and hand on this sort of thing. And how long am I going to be able to work? Who will employ me? Word gets round fast in psychiatry. I suppose the whole hospital was humming about me. And now everyone will be watching me, to see if I laugh too loudly, talk too much and too fast . . .'

She looked around the sitting-room, which was tidier than I had ever seen it, and said, 'When I was really bad I thought this place was "bugged" – did you know that? I thought a crowd of Fascists were after me. It was terrifying. I walked round the hospital one night and I met Kenny. He took me into his room and gave me tea, and when I told him about the bugging he gave me a sort of look, suspicious and wary. And he began to humour me. That's what they do with children, drunks and the very old: they humour them.'

I listened to her sad litany and tried to imagine what it

must be like. God knows I had seen enough patients to be able to empathize, but her degree of melancholy was of a different dimension, impossible to share and, because of that, unbearable for the individual overcome by it.

'Does Dave Hedley know about how you feel, Harriet?'

Surely Dave wouldn't have let her come on duty like this? A rather sly look came into her eyes, and she reminded me that she had always been a very good actress.

I said firmly, 'Well, don't come in tomorrow, will you.'

I would contact Dave and get him to come over and see her; and maybe Rosie would come up and try to persuade her to go down with her to the cottage.

'It's better for me if I come into the hospital. I don't want to be here on my own. Oh, Auntie Madge tries, but she doesn't know what to say to me, and I think she thinks that I might attack her or take off my clothes and run around screaming. Come and see me again soon.'

At least she wanted me to come again: I hung on to that as I went out. At the door I turned and said, 'Roger will come and see you, too. And Rosie.'

'That will be nice.'

Auntie Madge fluttered around me on the way out.

'Very down, isn't she? Always a sensitive girl, though. I used to think to meself "That girl's just like Mollie" — that was her mother, and she always used to suffer from her nerves. Spent half her life in hospital, she did. I used to be ever so sorry for Jim, Harriet's father . . . Pity he's not alive now. 'Course, she shouldn't ever have taken up this line of work, should she? Ever so trying. Doesn't eat, neither, just picks. Sits there not doing anything. It's not right, is it? I don't know what to do, I'm sure.'

When I got back to my house, I rang Dave Hedley but his wife said he had a very bad cold and had just gone off to sleep, so I told her not to bother waking him. What could he do? Harriet had someone with her after all, and although my first thought had been that she wasn't fit for duty I thought again of the misery of just sitting in the house and decided that at least she would have more company in the hospital.

I was awakened early by the telephone. I wasn't really surprised. It was Dave Hedley, his voice rough with laryngitis.

'Harriet's dead. She got up during the night and swallowed twenty barbiturate tablets. Could you go over right away?'

CHAPTER TWENTY

The curtains were drawn over the windows in Harriet's house. When Auntie Madge opened the door to me she looked pale but composed. I remembered that she had told me of one year in her life when her old father, her husband and a son of twelve had all died within months of each other, so she was well used to death. She showed me in to the darkened sitting-room, still unusually tidy, and said that the police had been informed and were on their way.

Auntie Madge had given Harriet a cup of coffee, and they had gone to bed at eleven o'clock, an hour after I had returned home. At about one, there was a sound of someone moving on the landing, and Harriet had called out that she was going to the lavatory and to go back to sleep. Waking out of a deep sleep at six o'clock, Auntie Madge had got up and, feeling anxious, she just didn't know why, she had looked in on Harriet; and going up to her, had found her dead.

'She must have taken these . . . They were beside her, on the table . . .'

Auntie Madge held up a bottle, which was quite empty. The label said that it had contained twenty Nembutal tablets, quite the strongest of the barbiturate group.

'I didn't know she took sleeping tablets. She told me she had been able to do without them since her treatment in hospital.'

'Did she leave a note or anything?'

'There was nothing. I'm in a daze . . . I can't believe it. Would you like some tea?'

I said I would. I didn't feel like anything but I thought it would give Auntie Madge something to do.

The sight of what she thought she might become had been

too much for Harriet. She had ruminated on that psychotic woman in the back ward and decided to take this quick way out of a situation which was too much for her, rather than live out her days under the shadow of impending madness. She knew that she would never be the same again, that even if her brain came back to moving as surely and as fast as ever (and nobody could reassure her that it would) no one could say for how long she would remain well. Along with sex, her cerebral apparatus meant so much to Harriet that to feel it crumbling was unbearable.

As with every suicide, I blamed myself. I went over all the causes and the explanations and the reasons, and I castigated myself for not staying with her last night, for not trying to get through to her better. I knew that I might have prevented her taking her life for a while, but could I have affected the ultimate outcome?

'Too clever, that's what she was. But it's so sad, a young girl with her life before her.' Auntie Madge came in with a tray, and after pouring us both a cup of tea she sat down in a chair and dabbed her eyes. I knew she was expecting me to weep, but I couldn't force one tear.

I said that I would like to see Harriet, when I had finished the scalding tea, and Auntie Madge sighed, put away her handkerchief and said to follow her.

On entering the bedroom you might have thought that Harriet was sleeping, until you went closer and saw that she was blue. She lay with her hands beside her in the tiny bed, her hair dark against the white sheet and the high-necked ruffled blue nightgown making her look very young. But her skin was assuming that ugly mottled cyanosed look that was a symptom of an overdose of barbiturate drugs.

I thought of other corpses I had seen. In Ireland if a person died, especially in tragic circumstances, there would be candles, prayers and flowers, with a constant procession of people creeping in and out of the room, to weep and kneel down and pray beside the body.

I dropped on my knees and said a prayer beside Harriet's stiff, lonely remains, and I imagined I could hear the old piercing shout and thought of her dashing along the hospital corridors with her hair and skirt flying. I looked at the peaceful remote expression on her face, and it seemed that perhaps this was the best way. It was a way that I could never take because I lacked the courage, but then, if I had been Harriet and knew that I was like someone whose internal batteries have gone and may never return, and if I woke at three in the morning and thought of my future, who knew how I might behave if I had the means of a painless way out?

There was a ring at the front door, and Auntie Madge went out with her skirts rustling.

'It's the police, I expect. Oh, I feel ever so bad that they have to come. Still, it's the law, isn't it? That's what Dr Hedley said when I rang him . . .'

I could hear Hedley's voice in the hall, and then he came up.

'This is a bad business.' He looked tired and toxic and his voice was rasping.

Auntie Madge made more tea, and while we waited for her to bring it in we went over what had happened during the past night. I felt sorry for Hedley, almost more than he felt guilty with himself. To any psychiatrist suicide of a patient means that you haven't really been able to persuade them that life is preferable to death. This feeling is often illogical and unfair, because anyone who really wants to die will ultimately find the means to do so, in spite of all possible support and help. Grief and shame on the psychiatrist's part are often due to his own ego being bruised by the patient's public confession that treatment has been·a failure. I felt like comforting Hedley by saying that maybe it was for the best: what was before Harriet, anyway, but the perpetual fear of a breakdown, and a lonely old age probably spent in an institution? I didn't do so because I knew his views as a Catholic on suicide and abortion.

'Could she have got up and taken too many pills after making herself woozy on one dose? It's pretty common, isn't it? You know, a person doesn't *really* want to die, but they do it by mistake.'

I held out a hopeful suggestion to Hedley, who rubbed his unshaven cheeks and looked at me out of bloodshot eyes.

'I doubt it. But let's hope the Coroner takes that view. Here are the police.'

The three policemen were large men, who tried to go up the stairs as gently as possible. Auntie Madge followed them with fearful eyes from the hall.

The phone went for Hedley and he said in a tired way that somebody wanted him at the hospital. Could I be available, as they'd probably need me at the inquest?

I went to the window of the sitting-room and watched him get into his car. He had always looked so clean and perky that it was odd to see him with stubble on his chin and an old polo-neck jersey instead of his bow tie. All of a sudden I had an intimation of how he would look as an old man, thin and shrivelled.

There was a noise on the stairs and Auntie Madge came in to say that they were taking Harriet away. She was being trundled down the stairs in a sort of canvas bag. Her thin feet stuck out obscenely, blue and blotched, but the toenails had the remnants of silver polish.

'Poor kid. Young to be a doctor, isn't she?' The policeman who said it was young, too, with a narrow pink face and a wispy moustache.

The body would lie in the police morgue now, awaiting the pathologist's knife.

I was glad to be kept busy at the hospital for the rest of the day, although everywhere I went they were talking about Harriet, and I was told that Sister Eccles was sitting in her office weeping, after having been given a sedative. I rang Rosie, to find that she had gone away for a week.

I didn't know whether anyone had told Roger, so I went up to his ward to do so. Milligan came out of the kitchen, carrying a cup of coffee, and said when she saw me, 'Oh, isn't it awful about Dr Bentley? I hear she was found dead. Was it . . . ?'

She wavered, seeing my face, and decided not to continue. Roger came out and beckoned me in to the office.

'I met Singh and he told me Harriet's dead. Is it true?'

I said that it was, and he looked out of the window at a

grey building opposite, where there were still bars on the windows, relics of the old custodial days.

'Such a tragedy, but you know I can't say I'm surprised. What could anyone do for her? It makes me laugh, all this fashionable claptrap about environment and a therapeutic atmosphere. We're the product of our genetic inheritance and Harriet had a loaded one. She knew the score: that she would break down again and again, each time more severely and becoming more and more reduced mentally, and she couldn't bear it. She had great courage, don't you think? She never wanted to grow old, and now she hasn't.'

Roger cleared his throat and began to stir his coffee vigorously. His words about Harriet were obviously sincere, and it was so unusual for Roger to find nice things to say about another human being, especially an individual so remote from his own background and personality as Harriet, that I was struck dumb.

'I suppose there'll have to be an inquest and all that sort of thing . . . Messy. No relatives, I hear, except a dim aunt? And poor you, you'll have to attend the inquest, I take it?'

'Yes.'

'Oh, the Coroner's decent – that's one boon in Haxton. He'll lean over backwards to get a "Death by Misadventure" verdict. It's much better than a "Suicide" one, especially if you're insured. A great many policies don't cover taking your own life. Gracious, think of the way she did it, getting up and coolly swallowing the tablets. Nothing sloppy . . . And she made a good job of it. A great many women attempt suicide and don't do it properly.' Roger's tone was almost admiring. 'Of course, all of us in this game have seen enough suicides to know how it should be done.'

'Yes, we get good Commando training,' I said. 'No wonder psychiatrists have the highest suicide rate amongst doctors.'

'And barbiturates are such a *clean* way. Not like wrist-slashing or throwing yourself in the river.'

He could have been talking about the best way to put in central heating and I thought of Harriet's poor blue feet rubbing against the banister, and the way her body was trundled down in the canvas bag as though it were a bale of hay.

Roger looked at me and then said, peering again out of the window, 'But I wish she hadn't done it, you know. Damn it, there's always a sporting chance, no matter how we comfort ourselves by saying she's better out of it. I couldn't kill myself because of the possibility of things changing. We'll miss her . . .'

Fortunately the inquest was held a few days later and the Coroner, a stout man with rimless glasses and sympathetic eyes, didn't ask me too much and brought in his verdict, that the death was a tragic one caused by Dr Bentley not having remembered how many tablets she had actually taken, and in a moment of confusion swallowing an overdose.

The verdict that the death was 'Misadventure' appeared in the local paper, and I had a job to hold off some curious reporters.

'Vultures!' Roger hissed, when I told him of the Press interest. 'Of course, the sudden death of a young and attractive doctor has all the elements of a scoop.'

Harriet was cremated two days after the inquest, and she would have hated the stilted little ceremony held at a crematorium, which reminded me of Waugh's *The Loved One*. Syrupy organ music provided a soporific background, and an unctuous clergyman made the most of an opportunity to talk in a voice reminiscent of a third-rate actor indulging in melodrama. The hospital was represented by myself, Hedley (still choking with a cold), Roger, Singh and Sister Eccles, who looked more like a distracted clown than ever.

When the flower-laden coffin disappeared behind the white and gold curtains, and everybody joined self-consciously in a hymn, I could hear and see Harriet guffawing loudly and making fun of the clergyman's prominent Adam's apple.

Roger came up to me as we were leaving the building. He looked immaculate in his dark suit and tie.

'God, how awful! Did you think Mrs Hedley looked grotesque? Drink or drugs? Talking of drink, I don't imbibe but there *are* times when one needs an anaesthetic. Let's go and have a glass of sherry. Did you notice Singh combing his hair before the ceremony? Typical! No sign of Mason. Probably droning on to some dim patient.'

I told Roger that I couldn't have a drink because I was on my way to Madley Clinic, for the last time, as it happened, because Ellison would be back next week. At this Roger congratulated me warmly. 'You'll be well shot of *that* chore,' he exclaimed.

It was quite unreasonable to feel so annoyed at the return of Ellison, and to know that after today I would have severed my connection with Madley. As I drove towards the hospital the weather outdid itself in beastliness. The wind drove the rain against the windows, so that the windscreen wipers made feeble, defeated swishes, and I had to turn on the car lights.

Mrs Sweetman gave me a few minutes to take off my coat and try and dry my wet and flattened hair, before she came in with the list of patients. She turned on the lights while I sat down carefully, keeping well away from the hole in the floor which the carpenters still hadn't fixed.

'The first patient is a boy of nine, Doctor, Roy Sears.'

Roy was a chubby boy with bright brown eyes, who came in accompanied by his mother, who was a midwife.

'What's the trouble, Mrs Sears?'

'Well, it sounds daft . . . I don't quite know how to tell you about it . . .'

'Would Roy like to tell me?'

But Roy, overcome by bashfulness, grew fiery red and stared desperately out of the window, which was one grey wet sheet.

I looked down at the GP's letter, which was very brief and said that Roy had been getting some 'queer turns' lately, and that his mother was concerned about him.

'What about these "turns", Mrs Sears?'

'Well, that's it. I mean, Roy's a good boy, doing well at school and never been really ill till he started to go like this. He looks a bit blank, his colour changes, and last week when he got one he came into the kitchen while I was making the supper and he said to me – well, go on, tell the lady what you told me you had turned into, Roy.'

Roy shuffled his feet and said, 'A biscuit.'

Mrs Sears was a nice little woman with the same bright eyes as her son, and she said in a worried voice, 'He told me he thought he'd turned into a fig roll biscuit. Five minutes later he'd forgotten and was all right. What could it be? His father's very worried.'

I rang the hospital at Bushy Park and arranged for Roy to have a brain recording, telling Mrs Sears that the attacks might be due to Roy's brain being overexcitable. I avoided the word 'epilepsy', although the attack sounded epileptiform in nature.

The next patient was a cross miner, who suffered from impotence and whose wife was making eyes at a silver-tongued navvy. Reassurance that the more he worried, the worse the impotence would become, plus a promise that I would write to his doctor and prescribe some male hormone tablets, sent him on his way not happy but consoled, and then I saw a little old woman who had had palpitations for five years. Nobody had found out why, and she looked very spry and lively for her seventy years. As she was getting up to go, she said something about 'The Irish Whip', and the penny dropped for me. Did she watch wrestling on TV every Saturday? Of course she did. Why hadn't she told anybody? With a sweet smile, she said that nobody had ever asked her! Then she must stop watching, I said: wrestling was too exciting for hearts that weren't as young as they used to be. Oh, that would be impossible, she said. Wrestling was the highlight of her week: couldn't I give her something for her palpitations so that she could view? We arrived at a compromise in which she promised to watch for only half an hour and I told her I would order a mild tranquillizer.

For ages I wondered why the name of the next patient was familiar: Phyllis Denning? Then I remembered that Mrs Redmond had mentioned that she wanted me to go and see her. The slender woman who sat in front of me had piercingly bright grey eyes and a way of looking sideways that gave her an oddly birdlike look. She had been a patient in Bushy Park for a short period five years ago. She didn't really know why but she had kept well ever since. The only time the doctor was called was to see her husband; she herself didn't bother with doctors. Her mother had left her some very good recipes for home medicines.

'Mr Denning's stomach is always getting upset.' She smoothed down the skirt of her trim suit with fluttering white hands. ''Course, he drinks so much. Last week he had a bad time with his stomach ... In bed for six weeks, he's been.'

How did she and her husband get on? I wondered about this from the tinkling laugh she gave when she spoke about him.

'Very badly.' She laughed again. They had never really had anything in common. She liked sewing and music and he only cared about his work and beer.

'Why don't you leave him?'

'Oh, he earns a good wage. He doesn't give me enough money sometimes, but I am able to get it.'

'How?'

'I have my means.' The little giggle again. 'I have my means ...'

Why had she come to the clinic? I asked. Apart from an odd fey quality about her she seemed perfectly sane.

Because Mr Denning kept saying that she was mad and that she'd have to go back to the mental hospital. She wanted to be able to say that the doctor had said she was *not* mad.

The room seemed dark even though I had the lights on, and what with the rain slashing against the window outside and Mrs Denning's high-pitched giggle, I began to sense a very odd quality about her. What were her husband's stomach upsets? She said that the doctor didn't know what to make of them. Supposing she was slowly poisoning him? I had a mental picture of her brewing her 'home remedies' in the kitchen of her cottage, giving that eerie laugh while her fat husband groaned upstairs.

When I told her that she most certainly wasn't mad, she got up and drew her coat around her.

Did I go home by the new bridge? she asked at the door. I said yes, I did, it was much the quickest way.

'I wouldn't go that way tonight. Not if I was you ...'

Before I had time to ask her why, she was gone.

The clinic was over at half-past six, by which time Mrs Sweetman had left and the worst of the traffic rush was over. The rain had stopped and the wind had died down, and as I drove towards Madley I had a good mind to give the new bridge a miss. It wouldn't take too long to go an alternative way. Then I thought that this was a matter of principle. If we took notice of everything bizarre that patients told us . . . Phyllis Denning was an eccentric who might equally have warned me about crossing water, or a Dark Stranger.

I drove with exquisite care to the set of traffic lights that came just before the bridge, and looking well to each side, I pressed the accelerator when the lights turned to green. Inching forward, I became sickeningly conscious that a lorry had appeared on my left, from nowhere, and seemingly out of control. I rammed down the brake and the lorry hurtled past me, missing me by a hair's breadth.

I thought my heart would jump out of my ribcage; my hands were so set that the wheel slithered through them. When I drew in to the side to look for a hankie, I found that my bag wasn't there, so I turned and drove back to the hospital. I was still shaking when I arrived.

There was a light on in the waiting-room, and when I went in there was no mistaking the huddled figure sitting on one chair with his feet up on another.

'Slightly late . . . an indisposition.' Mr Brooker's hat was on the back of his head like a halo, and his eyes were bleary. A smell of whisky wafted through the room.

'It's after seven and I'm on my way home, Mr Brooker,' I said. I went in to the clinic room and got my handbag.

'Lucky you *have* a home,' Mr Brooker said reproachfully when I came out. 'Not like me. House cold and bloody dogs yapping everywhere.'

I was very tired. The incident with the truck had frightened me and I had missed saying goodbye and thanks to Mrs Sweetman.

I looked around the dark old building with the stained walls and the familiar smell of must, disinfectant and human bodies. In the distance I could hear the Matron roaring at some unfortunate nurse. What would happen to the Taskers, with the fat white baby? And Cedric, would he survive in a hostile world? Could Vicky ever get over her moods?

'Oh, well, I know when I'm not welcome.' Mr Brooker had

probably heard the Matron, too, and didn't want to tangle with her. He gathered himself together and stood up with drunken dignity.

'You could at least smile at me, Doctor. Smile at me, *I'm lonely.*'

'And so am I, Mr Brooker,' I said, rushing out before he could cash in on my emotion.

This time I was well over the new bridge before I realized where I was.